HUMAN ANATOMY AND PHYSIOLOGY, PRACTICAL BOOK (BP107P)

Rajesh Kumar Mukherjee,
Dr. Dilip Kumar Roy.

First printing edition, 2024
Distribution rights to all territories (Worldwide rights)

ISBN 13: 978-93-341-0378-6

Dedication

This book is completely devoted to those individuals (Students) who continuously struggle to compete in this competitive world with truth by following the right path, don't try to harm others and try to live peacefully.

Most of the people during their challenging periods of life are self-constrict themselves and we the authors of this book striving to surpass our limits and present our achievements in the form of this book to everyone who aspires to improve themselves and enhance their abilities and knowledge of anatomical and physiological aspects in human being.

Regular expressions of gratitude or encouragement can significantly improve someone's life in a unique and elevated manner.

Thank You Everyone.

Content page

About the authors

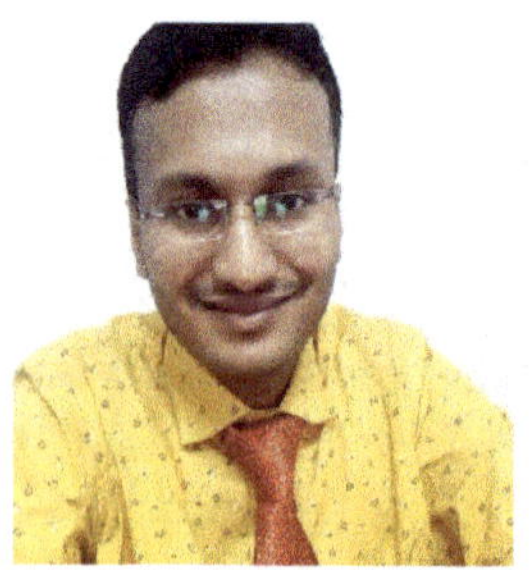

Mr. Rajesh Kumar Mukherjee, a Research Scholar (pursuing Ph.D. in Pharmacology from JIS University, Kolkata, West Bengal, India), has 3.10 years of industrial experience (R&D Analytical Development Laboratory and Pharmacovigilance) and 3.8 years of academic experience (currently working as an Assistant Professor in Brainware University, Department of Pharmaceutical Technology, Barasat, West Bengal, India). He has published 2 books, 2 patents, and a and a few research articles in reputed journals and secured lots of oral and poster presentation awards at the national and international levels.

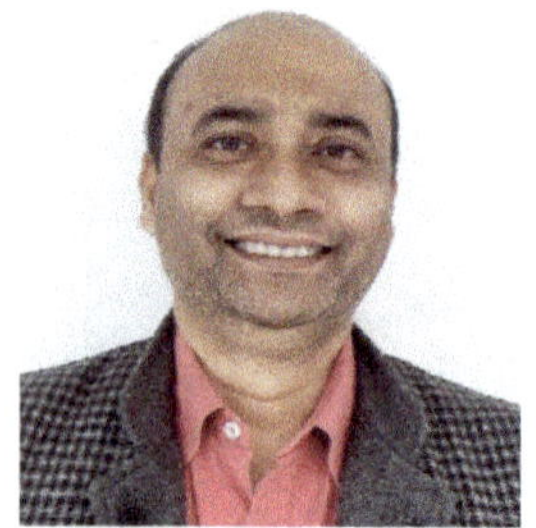

Dr. Dilip Kumar Roy, M. Pharm, Ph. D. from Jadavpur University, has renounced expertise for around 18 years in the Pharma and Biotech Industries (R&D) and 3+ years of academic experience (currently working as an Associate Professor at JIS University, Department of Pharmaceutical Technology, Kolkata, West Bengal, India). He has published more than 10+ review and research articles in reputed journals, 4+ books, and patents to his credit, secure awards in national and international levels, as well as guided a lot of Ph. D., M. Pharm, and B. Pharm students.

How to write any practical systematically?

(Please check this page below)
(what we teachers expected from students in their practical book)

Experiment Number – 01 or 02 ..

Topic of the Experiment

Aim: To study "the topic of experiment."

References: (Check the theory and practical from university/ college library and write at least 2 references in each experiments, inside each practical they are kept blank just we want you to check books in library and other platforms like internet to upgrade your knowledge levels)

1. Author full last name and first and second name initials after that, "book name", publication name if any, volume in roman letters, edition, year, page number.
Include which data are available for that particular book. e.g.,
2. Mukherjee R.K., Roy D.K. "Human Anatomy and Physiology, Practical Book (BP107P)", 1st Edition, 2024, Page No. 5-7.

Requirements:
a. Chemicals: (If any use in this practical).
b. Apparatus: (If any use in this practical).
c. Instruments: (If any use in this practical).
d. Directly write name if anything only for demonstration purpose for e.g., Human skeletal system, or any model or charts by which we learn.

Theory: All the theoretical data available in books related to that topic should be systematically written down. Avoid making mistakes, and if you do make a mistake in writing, simply correct it in a single stroke of line. Avoid using highlighters and use pens of blue or black colour, preferably ballpoint pens.

Procedure:
1. Point wise write down every step which you perform.
2. Write down the points in present tense because by which you read and perform your experiments.

Observation: If any particular observations are there like colour change, any movements and any such things are there by which you can conclude the things happen around in that practical.

Result: "was to be studied and performed" (mostly preferred word added in the result) it must be in past tense, any final reading after calculation must be placed in result section.

(Keep in mind if any diagrams, figures, flowcharts, tables and calculations are there then must be placed in the blank white pages).

Few Important Tips: As good habit.

1. Put your practical in your bag a day before practical perform.
2. Be happy: Because if you are happy and sound well, you connect with the environment, and results lead to a series of positive outcomes.
3. Eat well: Most of the practical's are blood related, so it's very important to eat well to prevent fainting, vertigo, and illness.

Inside laboratory:

1. Do gowning process wear lab coats (aprons), surgical caps, surgical mask, specs, surgical gloves and shoe covers (as per industry norms: GLP "Good Laboratory Practices").
2. Read thoroughly the lab manual or standard operating procedure for using any instrumentation or experiments after that you touch and perform the particular experiment and get better results.
3. Maintain cleanliness in working areas to prevent pathogens to enter in your body.
4. Carefully handle staining agents, acids, other chemicals and instruments so you are safe and tidy.
5. After completion of experiments put everything in proper places from where you take any apparatus or instruments so the later practical's you perform systematically.

[**Important note:** In the few sections of experimental procedure the 2nd part of procedure is which are performed earlier days beyond 2012, but after that Indian Pharmacy council decided to ban it because of certain reasons its clearly mentioned in the notice published in 19th January 2012, reference no. 10-1/2010-PCI Pt.1/4070442813 with the subject title "Alternative experiment model as per guidelines of CPCSEA and clearly stated that in point 1 and 2.

&

Similarly mentioned under prevention of cruelty to animal act (PCA) 1960, rule 16 (d).]

(The alternative procedures might be any simulation software's like: as reference
i. Human anatomy and physiology: BioDigital, Anatomy 3D Atlas, virtual physiology.
ii. Cell simulation: Vcell and other compartmental modelling softwares.
iii. Animal cell and tissue related simualions: Expharm, MyCalPharm.
iv. Docking (Protein ligand binding) software's: PKsim, discovery studio, Schrodinger.
v. Data-bases: pubchem, for protein- RCSB PDB, for genes- national genome data center.)

<u>Experiment Number – 01</u>

Study of compound microscope

<u>**Aim:**</u> To study the compound microscope.

<u>**References:**</u>
1.

2.

<u>**Requirements:**</u>
a. Apparatus: The specimens of cell/ tissue.
c. Instruments: The compound microscope.

<u>**Theory:**</u>
The compound microscope is a powerful optical instrument used to magnify small objects that are not visible to the naked eye. It consists of multiple lenses, which work together to achieve high levels of magnification. The theory behind the functioning of a compound microscope is based on the principles of optics and the behaviour of light.

This is one of the most commonly used instruments in medical, paramedical, and clinical laboratories. Researchers use it to study cell morphology, histology, histopathology, and microbiology.

A. Description of compound microscope: The compound microscope consists of the following primary components:
I. The supporting system.
II. The focusing system.
III. The optical or magnifying system.
IV. The illumination system, including: (a) A source of light. (b) Mirror. (c) Condenser.

I. The support system: Various functional units attach themselves to this framework. It consists of the following:
(a) Base: It is a heavy metallic, 'U'-shaped or 'horseshoe'-shaped base that supports the microscope on the work table and provides maximum stability.
(b) Pillars: Attached to the 'C'-shaped handle, two upright pillars extend upward from the base. This enables the tilting of the microscope at an appropriate angle for comfortable observation.

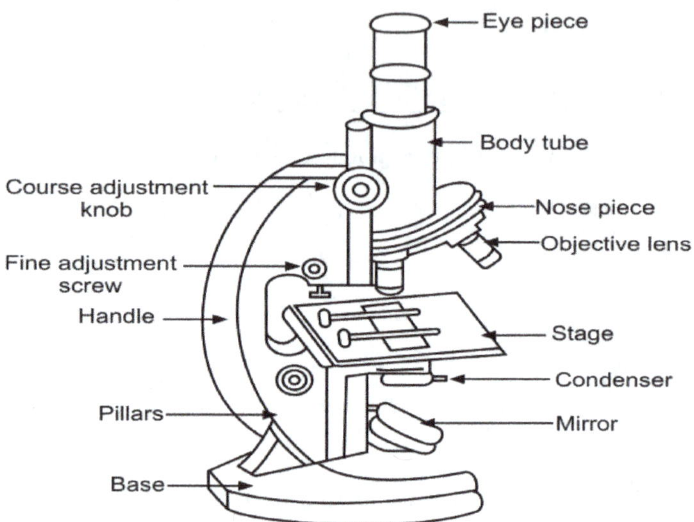

Fig. 1.1. The parts of compound microscope.

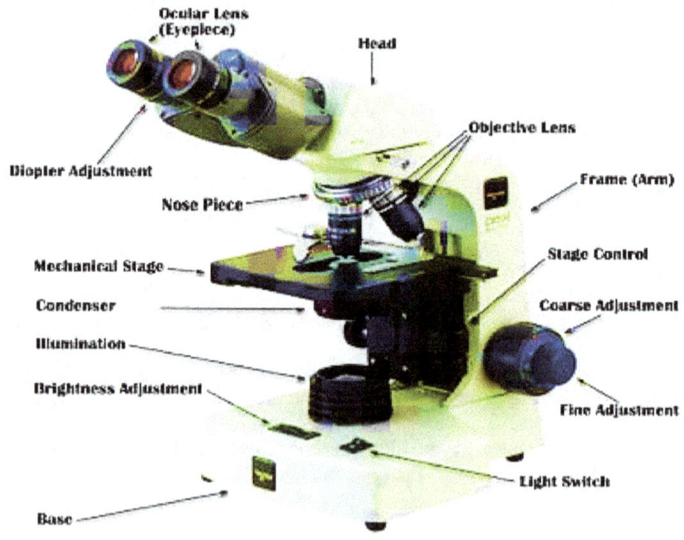

Fig. 1.2. The modern updated compound microscope.

(c) Body tube: Located at the upper end of the handle, this 16–17 cm long cylindrical tube is either vertical or angled, allowing light to pass through the eyepiece and into the observer's eye, thereby visualizing the image.

(d) The stage: This is a platform where the specimen slide is placed. The stage often comes with clips to hold the slide in place and mechanisms to move it precisely. The stage is a square platform with an aperture in its center and fitted to the limb below the objective lenses. When the slide is placed on it, converging rays of light emerging from the condenser pass through the slide and then the objective lens into the body tube. It can be either the fixed stage or the mechanical stage. The fixed stage has two clips that hold the slide in position. On the right side of the mechanical stage, there is a calibrated metal frame. It has a spring-mounted clip to hold the slide and two screw heads to move it from side to side, forward and backward. We also attach the vernier scale to indicate the degree of movement.

II. The focusing system: It includes both coarse and fine adjustments, utilizing screw heads to raise and lower the body tube for accurate slide focusing. The coarse adjustment operates similarly, requiring multiple rotations to move the tube over a short distance. It is employed for accurate focusing.

III. The optical or magnifying system: It consists of a body tube, an eyepiece, and the nose piece. The body tube is present between the upper end of the objective and eyepiece.

a. The eyepiece fits on top of the body tube, also known as ocular lens: This lens is positioned near the observer's eye. It magnifies the image produced by the objective lens. The eyepiece lens further enlarges the real image formed by the objective lens to produce a virtual image that the viewer can see. They can be 5X, 6X, 8X, 10X, or 15X. Each eyepiece has two lenses: the eye lens at the top and the field lens at the bottom. The field lens collects divergent rays, which are then passed through the eye lens to further magnify the image. The nose piece is made up of two parts: the fixed nose piece and the revolving nose piece. The fixed nose piece holds the revolving nose piece that carries interchangeable objective lenses.

b. The objective lenses are spring-loaded objectives of different magnifying powers. There are different types of objective lenses: low power objective (10X), high power objective (45X), oil immersion objectives (100X), and scanning objectives (3X). This is the lens closest to the specimen being observed. It typically has a short focal length and provides the initial magnification of the object. The objective lens creates a real, inverted, and magnified image of the object within the microscope tube.

Magnification: Magnification is the ability to make small objects appear larger, such as making a microscopic organism visible. The objective lenses magnify the images as stated below: The low power objective (10X) is equal to 10 x 10 = 100 times. We can calculate the high-power objective (45X) by multiplying 45 x 10 = 450 times. The goal for oil immersion is 100X, which is equivalent to 100 x 10 = 1000 times. The oil immersion (100X) objective features a very small aperture and a deep focusing position, precisely 1 mm from the slide. The right rays come from the objective's slide aperture, resulting in a faint image. Adding another medium to the slide, such as cedar wood oil, paraffin, or glycerine with the same refractive

index as glass, eliminates the thin air layer and creates a continuous medium. This avoids the refraction of light rays and results in a sharp image.

IV. The illumination system: A light source, usually a lamp or mirror, is used to illuminate the specimen from below, proper illumination or lighting is necessary for the microscope to function, the illumination system's goal is to provide uniform, soft, and bright illumination.

The illumination system consists of:
(a) Source of light: It may be external (natural day light, electric lamp, or tube light) or internal (electric in-built light source).
(b) A condenser is a system of lenses mounted on a short cylinder below the stage. This lens system is used to focus light onto the specimen. It is positioned below the stage and helps improve the clarity and contrast of the image.
(c) Mirror: Beneath the condenser, a double-sided mirror features a flat side and a concave side, allowing for rotation in all directions. It focuses light rays into a solid cone of light on the material under study and helps to resolve the image.
(d) Tube: The tube connects the eyepiece to the objective lens. It maintains the proper distance between these lenses, which is critical for accurate magnification and focusing.
(e) Iris diaphragm: Installed within a condenser, the Iris diaphragm is a thin, opaque membranous structure that features a small lever on its side. The lever can adjust the size of the diaphragm's aperture, allowing less or lighter to fall on the side.

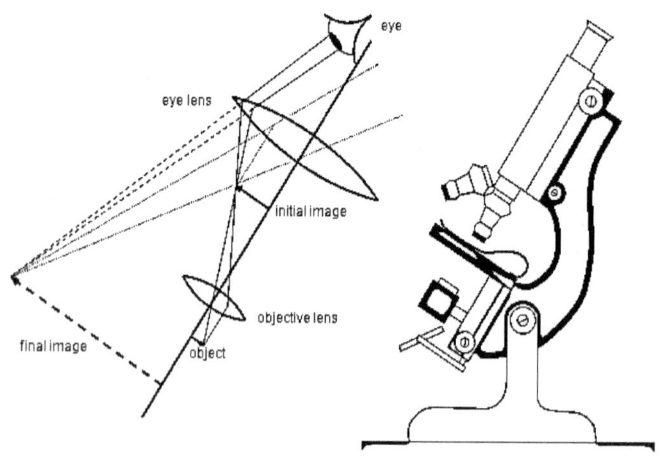

Fig. 1.3. Working principle of compound microscope.

Working principle: The compound microscope operates based on the principle of light refraction through lenses:
a. Light source and condenser: Light from the illumination system passes through the condenser lens, which focuses it onto the specimen, the light then passes through the specimen, gathering information about its structure.
b. Objective lens magnification: The objective lens, positioned close to the specimen, collects the light that has passed through the specimen and forms a magnified real image. This image is inverted due to the nature of lens refraction.
c. Magnification by the eyepiece: The real image formed by the objective lens is then magnified further by the eyepiece lens. This lens produces a virtual image that appears much larger to the observer. The overall magnification of the microscope is the product of the magnifications of the objective lens and the eyepiece.
d. Image formation: The observer looks through the eyepiece and perceives a large, detailed image of the specimen. The combined optical system allows for the magnification and resolution necessary to observe fine details that would be impossible to see with the naked eye.

Function: It performs the following functions like:
i. Magnification: The compound microscope uses a combination of two sets of lenses—objective lenses and the eyepiece (ocular lens)—to magnify the specimen. The objective lens, located near the specimen, creates an enlarged image. The eyepiece then further magnifies this image, allowing the observer to see the object in great detail.
ii. Resolution: One of the critical functions of a compound microscope is to improve the resolution, which is the ability to distinguish between two closely spaced points. Higher resolution enables the microscope to reveal fine structural details of the specimen that would otherwise be invisible to the naked eye.
iii. Illumination: The microscope includes a light source or mirror that illuminates the specimen from below. This lighting is essential for observing transparent or semi-transparent samples. The light passes through the specimen, making its features more visible and easier to study.
iv. Contrast enhancement: Compound microscopes often use a condenser lens to focus light on the specimen and enhance contrast. This allows for better differentiation between various structures within the specimen. Some microscopes also have filters or use stains to improve contrast, making it easier to observe specific parts of the specimen.
v. Detailed examination of specimens: The microscope allows for a detailed examination of biological samples, such as cells, tissues, and microorganisms. It is widely used in fields like biology, medicine, and research to study cell structures, identify pathogens, and analyse complex biological processes.
vi. Documentation and analysis: Many modern compound microscopes are equipped with digital cameras or imaging systems that allow users to capture images or videos of the specimens. This functionality is crucial for documentation, analysis, and sharing findings with other researchers or students.

Practical use: Compound microscopes are widely used in biology, medicine, and research. They enable scientists to observe cells, bacteria, and other micro-organisms, as well as tissue structures, at high magnifications.

Procedure:
Procedure of compound microscope are as follows:
a. Clean the compound microscope with clean and clear cotton cloth.
b. Prepare carefully the slides or take the pre-prepared specimens of cell/ tissue.
c. Turn on the light source of the microscope/ adjust the microscope mirror correctly where you get proper light.
d. Adjusting the microscope focus by using course and fine adjustment knob.
e. Higher magnification (if needed) use oil immersion (for 100x objective)
f. Recording observations: By drawing it in your note book you record your observations any significant features or details observed.
g. Capture images: If your microscope is equipped with a camera, take photographs or videos of the specimen for further analysis and documentation.
h. Turn off the light switch after completion.
i. Clean and store the microscope in a safe, dry place to prevent damage.

Observation: By knowing the parts and using the microscope one should understand how to handle it, by using the specimens (prepared slides) the stains or coloured shaped objects of different parts of any cell/ tissue in the slide are observed by the help of compound microscope.

Result: The compound microscope by using specimens was performed and the parts of microscope was to be studied.

<u>Experiment Number – 02</u>

Microscopic study of epithelial and connective tissue.

<u>**Aim:**</u> To study the microscopical evaluation of epithelial and connective tissue.

<u>**Reference:**</u>
1.

2.

<u>**Requirements:**</u>
a. Apparatus: The Specimen of epithelial and connective tissue.
b. Instrument: The compound microscope.

<u>**Theory:**</u>
A. Epithelial tissue: An epithelial tissue is a type of tissue composed of layers of cells that protect the surfaces of the body, line cavities, and constitute glands. The integumentary system functions as a protective barrier, safeguarding the body against the external surroundings and regulating the absorption and elimination of chemicals.
Structure:
a. Cell arrangement: The densely clustered epithelial cells, with reduced gaps between cells, help to the creation of a seamless layer. These cells are arranged in either single layers (the simple epithelium) or many layers (the stratified epithelium).

b. Cell shape: Cells exhibit a range of shapes, therefore facilitating their classification into distinct categories.
i. Squamous cells, which are present in the lining of blood arteries, are uniformly flat and thin.
ii. Cuboidal cells are cube-shaped cells found in the lining of the kidney tubule.
iii. Columnar cells are characterized by their towering stature and resemblance to columns, such as the endothelium of the gastrointestinal tract.

c. Polarity: Epithelial cells possess an apical surface exposed to the external environment or an interior cavity, together with a basal surface interconnected with a basement membrane.

d. Avascular: Epithelial tissue is devoid of blood vessels and depends on the release of nutrients and oxygen by diffusion from the connective tissues underneath it.

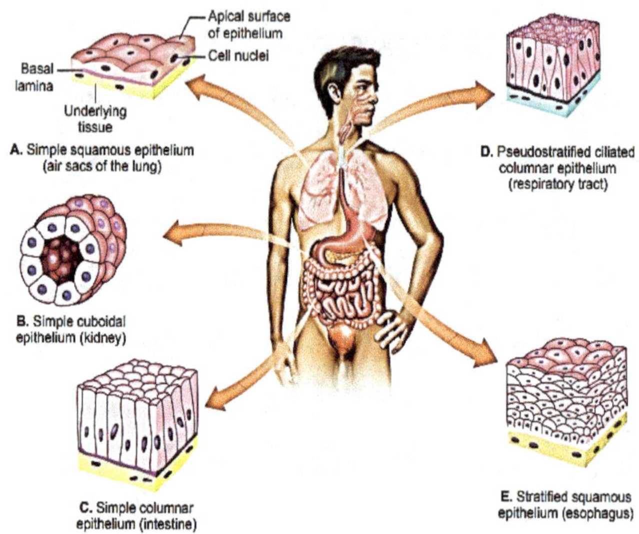

Fig. 2.1. Epithelial tissue.

Functions:

i. Protection: It functions as a protective barrier against physical, chemical, and biological strain and degradation, including skin injury.

ii. Absorption: Enhances the assimilation of nutrients and other compounds (e.g., intestinal mucosa).

iii. Secretion: Generates glands responsible for the secretion of hormones, enzymes, mucus, and other compounds (e.g., sweat glands).

iv. Excretion: Facilitates the removal of waste materials.

Sensory reception refers to the presence of sensory receptors, such as taste buds, that permit the detection of environmental changes.

B. Connective tissue: It is defined as the predominant and most varied form of tissue in the human body. It provides structural support, forms cohesive bonds, and protects tissues and organs. Compared to epithelial tissue, connective tissue generally has a smaller number of cells and a larger amount of extracellular matrix.

Structure:

I. Cells: This group encompasses a range of cell types, including fibroblasts responsible for fiber production, macrophages linked to immunological response, adipocytes engaged in fat storage, and mast cells involved in inflammatory response.

II. Extracellular Matrix (ECM): A mostly non-cellular constituent of connective tissue. It comprises:

a. Fibres:
i. Collagen fibers provide both structural integrity and support.
ii. Elastic fibers enable tissues to regain their initial form following elastic deformation.
iii. Reticular fibers: They establish interconnected networks of support.
iv. Ground substance: A gelatinous substance composed of water, glycosaminoglycans, proteoglycans, and glycoproteins that occupies the interstitial space between cells and fibrils.

Types of connective tissues:
a. Loose Connective Tissue: Characterised by a higher proportion of basement material and a lower number of fibers; encompasses areolar, adipose (fat), and reticular tissue.
b. Dense Connective Tissue: This tissue is characterized by a higher concentration of fibers and a lower amount of ground material. It encompasses dense regular tissue, such as tendons and ligaments, and dense irregular tissue, particularly the dermis.
c. The category of specialized connective tissue that encompasses cartilage, bone, blood, and lymph.

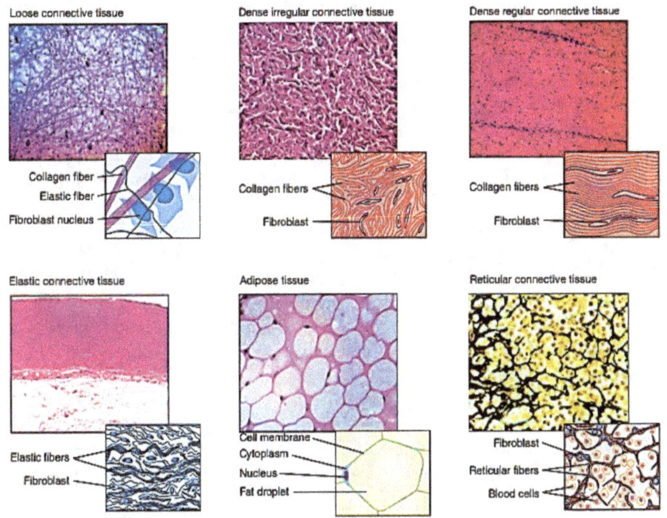

Fig. 2.2. Connective tissue.

Functions:
i. Support and structure: This is a systematic framework for organs and the entire body, encompassing bones and cartilage.
ii. Binding and connecting: This process facilitates the establishment of links between different tissues and organs. For example, tendons serve to link muscles to bones.
iii. Protection: The kidneys are enveloped by adipose tissue, which serves to cushion and safeguard the organs.
iv. Storage: The body stores energy as adipose tissue and minerals, including calcium present in bones.
v. Transport: Blood, a fibrous tissue, transports nutrients, gasses, and metabolic by-products.
The immune defence system comprises cells that combat illnesses and external invaders, such as white blood cells found in blood and lymphatic tissue.

Procedure:

I. Procedure for ready-made prepared specimens:
a. Clean the compound microscope with clean and clear cotton cloth.
b. Prepare carefully the slides or take the pre-prepared specimens of epithelium and connective tissue.
c. Turn on the light source of the microscope/ adjust the microscope mirror correctly where you get proper light.
d. Adjusting the microscope focus by using course and fine adjustment knob.
e. Recording observations: By drawing it in your note book you record your observations any significant features or details observed.
g. Capture images: If your microscope is equipped with a camera, take photographs or videos of the specimen for further analysis and documentation.
h. Turn off the light switch after completion.
i. Clean and store the microscope in a safe, dry place to prevent damage and same with the glass slide or tissue specimens.

II. Procedure for the actual thin tissue section withdrawn and prepare slides:
A. Sample collection and fixation:
i. Collecting the tissue sample: Obtain tissue samples using a biopsy, surgery, or dissection. Samples should be taken carefully to avoid damage to the tissue.
ii. Fixation: Immediately fix the tissue samples in a fixative solution (e.g., 10% formalin) to preserve their structure and prevent decay. Fixation hardens the tissue by cross-linking proteins, which helps maintain the morphology of the cells and extracellular components.

B. Tissue processing:
i. Dehydration: Immerse the fixed tissue in a series of ethanol solutions with increasing concentrations (e.g., 70%, 80%, 90%, and 100%). This removes water from the tissue.
ii. Clearing: Replace the ethanol with a clearing agent like xylene, which makes the tissue transparent and prepares it for infiltration with paraffin. iii. Embedding: Immerse the tissue in melted paraffin wax, which infiltrates the

tissue, replacing the xylene. Once embedded, allow the paraffin to solidify. This provides support for cutting thin sections.

C. Sectioning:
i. Cutting sections: Use a microtome to slice the paraffin-embedded tissue into thin sections, typically 4-6 micrometers thick, the thinness allows for light to pass through the sample for microscopic evaluation.
ii. Mounting: Carefully transfer the tissue sections onto glass microscope slides. This can be done by floating the sections on warm water and then placing them onto slides.

D. Staining:
i. Deparaffinization and hydration: Remove the paraffin wax by placing the slides in xylene and then rehydrate them through a series of decreasing ethanol concentrations (e.g., 100%, 90%, 80%, 70%) down to water. This prepares the tissue to accept stains.
ii. Staining: Apply stains to the tissue to highlight different structures, common stains include:
a. Haematoxylin and Eosin (H&E): Haematoxylin stains the nuclei blue-purple, while eosin stains the cytoplasm and extracellular matrix pink. This is the most common staining method for general tissue structure observation.
b. Periodic acid-Schiff (PAS): Stains carbohydrates and mucopolysaccharides, useful for detecting basement membranes and mucus.
c. Masson's Trichrome: Differentiates between muscle (red), collagen (blue or green), and cytoplasm (pink), making it valuable for connective tissue evaluation.
iii. Dehydration and clearing: After staining, dehydrate the slides again through increasing ethanol concentrations, clear with xylene, and prepare them for mounting.
iv. Mounting and cover slip.
v. Apply a drop of mounting medium (e.g., Canada balsam or synthetic resin) onto the tissue section on the slide.
vi. Place a coverslip over the tissue to protect the sample and improve optical quality.

E. Microscopical examination:
a. Using a Light Microscope: Begin with a low-power objective (e.g., 4x or 10x) to locate areas of interest, then switch to a higher power objective (e.g., 40x or 100x) for detailed examination.
b. Identify Tissue Types: i. Epithelial Tissue: Look for closely packed cells forming continuous sheets, with minimal intercellular space. Identify the shape of cells (squamous, cuboidal, columnar) and the number of layers (simple or stratified). ii. Connective Tissue: Identify the extracellular matrix, fibers (collagen, elastic, reticular), and different cell types (fibroblasts, macrophages, etc.). Note the density of the fibers and the presence of ground substance. c. Photomicrography: Capture images of the observed sections using a camera attached to the microscope, if available. These images can be used for further analysis, documentation, or presentations.

F. Disposal:
a. Biohazard waste: Dispose of unused tissue, gloves, and other disposable materials in biohazard containers following local regulations.

b. Disinfect work area: Clean and disinfect the work area and equipment to prevent contamination and infection.

G. Safety and ethical considerations:
i. Consent: Obtain informed consent from patients or appropriate ethical clearance for animal studies.
ii. Animal welfare: Follow guidelines for humane treatment of animals in research. (CPCSEA: The Committee for the Purpose of Control and Supervision of Experiments on Animals.) after committee hear and passes your form-B.

Observation: By knowing the parts of epithelial and connective tissue using the microscope one should understand the differences between them, by using the specimens (prepared slides) the stains or coloured shaped objects of different parts of tissue in the slide are observed by the help of compound microscope.

Result: The microscopical evaluation of epithelial and connective tissue by using specimens was performed under the microscope and the parts of this tissues was studied.

Experiment Number – 03

Microscopic study of muscular and nervous tissue.

Aim: To study the microscopical evaluation of muscular and nervous tissue.

References:
1.

2.

Requirements:
a. Apparatus: The Specimen of muscular and nervous tissue.
b. Instruments: The compound microscope.

Theory:
A. Muscular Tissue: Muscular tissue is composed of cells that are specifically adapted for the purpose of muscular contraction and force production. It is crucial in physiological processes such as bodily movement, posture maintenance, and heat generation.

Types of Muscular tissue: There are three primary categories of muscle tissue, each possessing unique attributes and performing specific roles:
i. Skeletal Muscle:
a. Structure: Skeletal muscle cells, or muscle fibers, are elongated, cylindrical, multinucleated, and striated (exhibiting a visible striping effect caused by the organization of actin and myosin filaments). The fibers are arranged in bundles enveloped by connective tissue.
b. Control: Skeletal muscles are under voluntary control, indicating that they are deliberately regulated by the neurological system.
c. Function: These muscles are connected to bones by tendons and contribute to skeletal movement (e.g., ambulation, item lifting). Furthermore, they assist in preserving posture and producing thermal energy during contraction.

ii. Cardiac Muscle:
a. Structure: Cardiac muscle cells follow the striated pattern of skeletal muscle, but they are shorter, branching, and linked together by intercalated discs. Located within these discs are gap junctions and desmosomes, which enable the coordinated contraction of the cardiac muscle.
b. Control: Cardiac muscle is subject to involuntary regulation by the autonomic nervous system and specific speed-regulating cells located within the heart.
c. Function: This particular muscle tissue is only located within the heart, where it undergoes regular contractions to facilitate the circulation of blood throughout the whole body.

iii. Smooth Muscle:

a. Structure: Smooth muscle cells bear a spindle-shaped morphology (tapered at both extremities), lack striated patterns, and possess a solitary nucleus. Unlike striated muscles, the organization of actin and myosin in these muscles is less structured, resulting in the absence of apparent striations.

b. Control: Smooth muscle is subject to involuntary regulation by the autonomic nerve system and hormone agents.

c. Function: Smooth muscle is present in the walls of hollow organs such as blood arteries, intestines, and bladder. It facilitates the regulation of blood circulation, food transit in the digestive system (peristalsis), and maintenance of airway diameter.

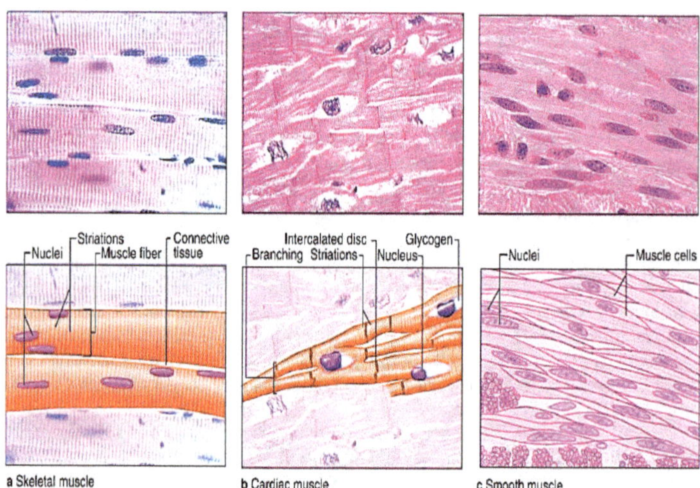

Fig 3.1. Muscle tissue.

Characteristics of Muscular tissue:

i. Excitability: The capacity to exhibit electrical impulses in response to stimuli such as nerve messages and hormones.

ii. Contractility: The capacity to contract vigorously when stimulated, hence facilitating movement.

iii. Extensibility: The ability to be stretched without sustaining injury.

iv. Elasticity: The capacity to regain its initial form following elongation or contraction.

B. Nervous Tissue: Nervous tissue is specialized for the mechanisms of communication and regulation. The central nervous system comprises neurons (nerve cells) and neuroglia (supporting cells) and is responsible for tactile perception, information processing, and signal transmission.

Constituents of Nervous Tissue:
I. Neurones:
a. Structure: Neurons are specialized cells consisting of three primary components:
Anatomical structure: Comprises the nucleus and organelles, serving as the core metabolic hub of the neuron, a dendrite is a brief, branching projection that receives impulses from neighbouring neurons or sensory receptors and transmits them to the cell body. An axon is an elongated neural structure that carries signals from the cell body to neighbouring neurons, muscles, or glands. An axon can be enveloped by a myelin sheath, produced by glial cells, which serves to insulate and accelerate the transmission of signals.

Cellular function: Neurons propagate electrical signals known as action potentials. Their role includes the processing of sensory information, regulation of muscles, and execution of intricate cognitive processes like thinking and remembering.

II. Neuroglia (Glial Cells): Neuroglia encompasses several types:
a. Astrocytes are spherical cells that offer structural and metabolic assistance to neurons, control the blood-brain barrier, and preserve the extracellular milieu.
b. Oligodendrocytes are responsible for the formation of the myelin coating around axons in the central nervous system (CNS).
c. In the peripheral nervous system (PNS), Schwann cells are responsible for the production of myelin.
d. Microglia: Function as immunological cells in the central nervous system, eliminating pollutants and contaminants.
e. Ependymal cells are tissue cells that line the cavities of the brain and spinal cord and aid in the circulation of cerebrospinal fluid.

Functional role: Neuroglia offers support and protection to neurons, regulates homeostasis, supplies nutrients, eliminates waste, and facilitates signal transmission.

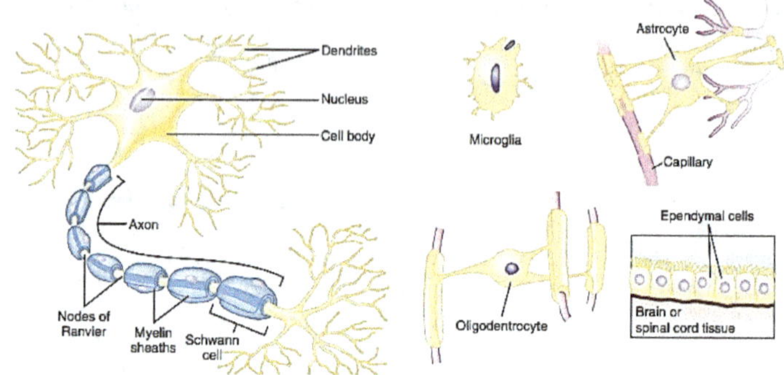

Fig. 3.2. Nervous tissue.

Characteristics of the nervous tissue:
Excitability refers to the intrinsic capacity of neurons to generate electrical impulses in response to stimulation, conductivity refers to the ability of neurons to propagate electrical impulses across long distances, therefore enabling communication across various regions of the body, integration refers to the process by which nerve tissue combines sensory input, interprets information, and coordinates suitable responses.

Functions of neuronal tissue:
i. Sensory Input: Neurons register alterations in the surroundings (either internal or external) by means of sensory receptors and transmit information to the central nervous system (CNS).
ii. Integration: The central nervous system (comprising the brain and spinal cord) receives and interprets sensory information, executes judgments, and produces reactions.
iii. Motor output: Motor neurons relay impulses from the central nervous system (CNS) to effector organs (muscles and glands) in order to trigger a reaction, such as the contraction of muscles or the release of hormones.
iv. Homeostasis: Nervous tissue regulates and coordinates bodily activities (such as heart rate, breathing, and digestion) to maintain homeostasis.
v. Cognitive function: Nervous tissue plays a role in complex cognitive processes like learning, memory, reasoning, and emotions.

<u>Procedure:</u>
I. Procedure for ready-made prepared specimens:
a. Clean the compound microscope with clean and clear cotton cloth.
b. Prepare carefully the slides or take the pre-prepared specimens of epithelium and connective tissue.
c. Turn on the light source of the microscope/ adjust the microscope mirror correctly where you get proper light.
d. Adjusting the microscope focus by using course and fine adjustment knob.

e. Recording observations: By drawing it in your note book you record your observations any significant features or details observed.

g. Capture images: If your microscope is equipped with a camera, take photographs or videos of the specimen for further analysis and documentation.

h. Turn off the light switch after completion.

i. Clean and store the microscope in a safe, dry place to prevent damage and same with the glass slide or tissue specimens.

II. Procedure for the actual thin tissue section withdrawn and prepare slides:

A. Preparation: For Muscle tissue

i. Gather equipment and materials: Ensure all necessary tools are sterilized and readily available, including scalpels, forceps, scissors, sterile gloves, syringes, fixatives, and containers for tissue samples.

ii. Sterilization: Clean the work area and sterilize instruments to prevent contamination. Wear sterile gloves and use aseptic techniques throughout the procedure.

iii. Labelling: Prepare and label containers for tissue samples with relevant information (e.g., patient ID, type of tissue, date, etc.).

B. Tissue collection: Muscle tissue

i. Anesthesia: If working with live animals or patients, administer appropriate anesthesia to minimize pain and discomfort.

ii. Incision: Make a precise incision over the area of interest using a sterile scalpel. For muscle biopsies, choose a site with minimal risk of complications.

iii. Tissue extraction: Carefully isolate and remove a small section of muscle tissue using forceps and scissors. Avoid damaging the surrounding structures.

iv. Hemostasis: Control any bleeding using sterile gauze, pressure, or cauterization if necessary.

v. Closure: If necessary, close the incision with sutures or surgical glue. Apply a sterile dressing to the area.

C. Preparation: For Nervous tissue

a. Craniotomy or laminectomy: In cases of nervous tissue extraction, such as brain or spinal cord, perform a craniotomy (removal of a portion of the skull) or laminectomy (removal of a section of the vertebral bone).

b. Tissue dissection: Use fine-tipped instruments to carefully expose and isolate the nervous tissue. Take care to avoid damaging surrounding blood vessels and nerves.

c. Tissue sampling: Gently extract a section of nervous tissue (e.g., biopsy of a brain tumor, spinal cord segment) using a micro dissecting tool. If working with brain tissue, ensure you're targeting the correct anatomical region.

d. Closure: Reconstruct the protective layers (e.g., dura mater) and close the surgical site, using sutures or staples as appropriate.

Tissue preservation:
i. Fixation: Immediately immerse the extracted tissue in a fixative solution (e.g., formaldehyde, glutaraldehyde) to preserve its structure. For some applications, snap-freezing in liquid nitrogen might be preferable.
ii. Labeling and storage: Place the fixed tissue in labeled containers and store it at the appropriate temperature, depending on the downstream analysis (e.g., histological examination, molecular studies).

Safety and ethical considerations:
i. Consent: Obtain informed consent from patients or appropriate ethical clearance for animal studies.
ii. Animal welfare: Follow guidelines for humane treatment of animals in research. (CPCSEA: The Committee for the Purpose of Control and Supervision of Experiments on Animals.) after committee hear and passes your form-B.

Observation: By knowing the parts of muscular and nervous tissue using the microscope one should understand the differences between them, by using the specimens (prepared slides) the stains or coloured shaped objects of different parts of tissue in the slide are observed by the help of compound microscope.

Result: The microscopical evaluation of muscular and nervous tissue by using specimens was performed under the microscope and the parts of this tissues was studied.

Experiment Number – 04

Identification of axial bones.

Aim: To study the identification of axial bones.

References:
1.

2.

Requirements: Human skeletal system.

Theory:
The axial skeleton is the central region of the body, one of the two primary divisions of the human skeletal system, alongside the appendicular skeleton. The axial skeleton functions as the central, structural framework of the body, offering support and protection to the organs and serving as a point of attachment for the appendicular skeleton, which encompasses the limbs.

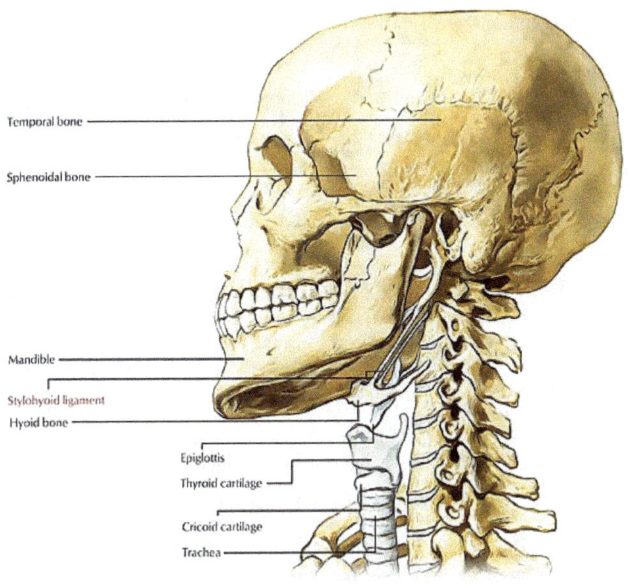

Fig. 4.1. Human cranium and facial bone.

Structure of the Axial skeleton: The axial skeleton is comprised of 80 bones, organized into three primary sections: the cranium, spinal column, and thoracic cage.

I. Cranial bone (22 bones): The skull consists of two primary components: the cranium and the face bones.

a. Cranium (8 skeletal bones):

i. The frontal bone (1 bone) is responsible for structuring the forehead and the top portion of the eye sockets.

ii. The parietal bones (2 bones) are situated on the lateral and superior aspects of the skull cranium regions.

iii. Temporal bones (2 bones) are located inferior to the parietal bones, it provides the anatomical framework for the ears.

iv. Occipital bone (1 bone) Comprises the posterior aspect of the skull and the inferior aspect of the cranium, encompassing the foramen magnum, a physical aperture through which the spinal cord connects with the brain.

v. Sphenoid bone (1 bone): A cartilaginous bone located in the inferior (beyond) parts of the cranium, which contributes to the cranial floor and the lateral parts of the skull.

vi. Ethmoid bone (1 bone): A superficial, porous bone situated in the space between the eyes, playing a role in the inner wall of the orbit, the nasal cavity, and the nasal septum.

b. Facial bones (it consists of 14 bones):
i. The nasal bones (2 bones) are twin small bones that constitute the bridge of the nose.
ii. The maxillae (2 bones) are the bone structures and uphold the upper jaw support the top teeth and are integral to the orbits and nasal cavity.
iii. The zygomatic bones (2 bones), collectively referred to as the cheekbones, are responsible for the elevation of the cheeks and a portion of the orbit.
iv. Mandible (1 bone), the mandible is the lower jaw bone, the sole mobile (moveable) bone in the head, which supports the lower teeth.
v. The lacrimal bones (2 bones), those are small bones that are embedded in the medial wall of each orbit and store and carry the lacrimal sac.
vi. The palatinate bones (2 bones), constitute the posterior portion of the hard palate as well as a portion of the nasal cavity and orbit.
vii. The inferior nasal conchae (2 bones) are slender, scroll-shaped bones that are integral components of the lateral walls of the nasal cavity.
vii. Vomer (1 bone) A slender, planar bone that constitutes the inferior section of the nasal septum.

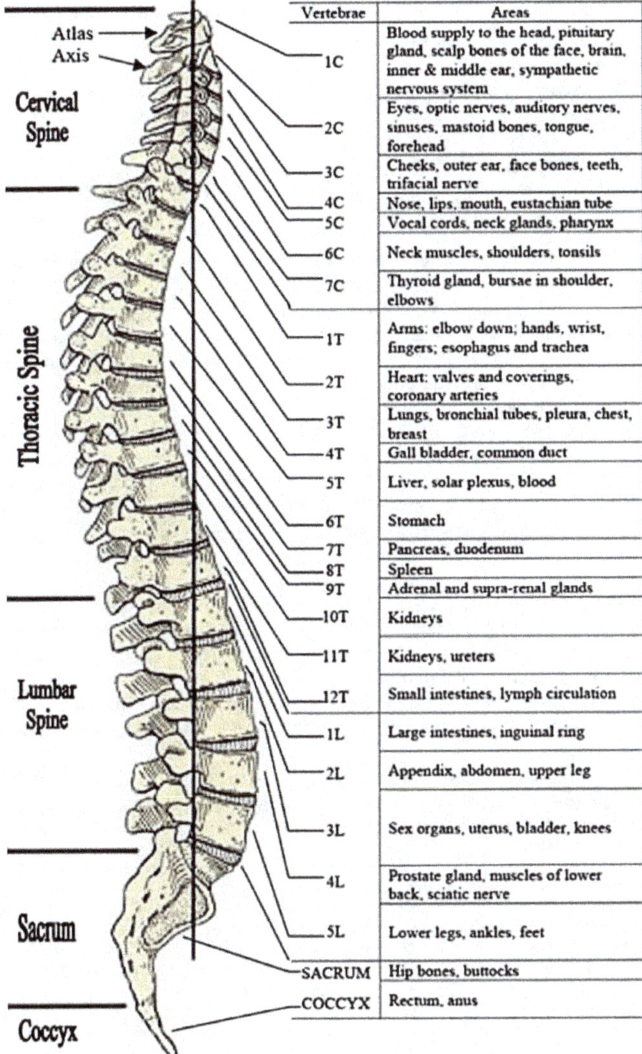

Fig. 4.2. Human vertebral column.

II. The vertebral column, often known as the spine, is a pliable spinal column consisting of 26 bones that stretch from the head to the pelvis. This is partitioned into five distinct regions:
A. Cervical vertebrae consist of seven bones: The vertebrae are situated inside the cervical area and are characterized by their diminutive size and low weight.
i. The C1 vertebra (Atlas) provides support to the skull and enables the normal nodding movement of the head.
ii. The C2 vertebra (Axis): It features like a bony projection known as the dens, enabling the head to undergo rotation.

B. The thoracic vertebrae consist of 12 bones: Placing itself in the upper and mid-back regions, each thoracic vertebra forms articulations with a pair of ribs, therefore providing support and protection for the thoracic organs.
i. Lumbar vertebrae (5 bones) those are located in the lumbar region, these vertebrae are comparatively bigger and more robust, specifically intended to support the load of the upper body.
a. Sacrum (1 bone formed by 5 fused vertebrae): The sacrum bone, a triangle bone located at the base of the spine, consists of five fused vertebrae and serves as a connection between the spine and the pelvis.
b. Coccyx (1 bone, formed by 4 fused vertebrae): The coccyx bone widely referred to as the tailbone, the coccyx is a compact, triangular bone made up of four fused vertebrae located for the attachment of ligaments and muscles of the pelvic   floor.

III. Thoracic cage (consisting of 25 bones): The thoracic cage, alternatively referred to as the rib cage, constitutes the structural skeleton of the chest, this structure comprises the sternum, ribs, and thoracic vertebrae.
i. Sternum (1 bone): The sternum, often known as the breastbone, is a planar metacarpal bone situated centrally in the chest. It is split into three sections:
a. Manubrium: The superior portion that forms an articulation with the clavicles (collarbones) and the first set of ribs.
b. Body: The elongated, central region, to which the majority of the ribs connect.
c. The Xiphoid Process is a diminutive cartilaginous projection located at the inferior aspect of the sternum, which undergoes ossification into bone as its ages.

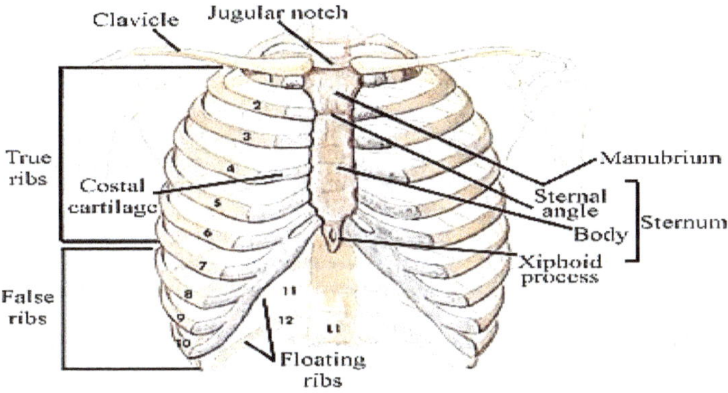

Fig. 4.3. Human rib cage.

ii. Ribs (24 bones): Each of the twelve pairs of ribs in the rib cage is connected posteriorly to the thoracic vertebrae.
a. The true ribs (1-7 bones): Each of the first seven pairs is connected to the sternum directly by costal cartilage.
b. The false ribs (8-10 bones): The next three pairs are connected to the sternum indirectly by means of the cartilage of the seventh rib.
c. The floating ribs (11-12): The last two pairs of ribs become detached from the sternum and are thus referred to as floating ribs. These structures offer protection to the kidneys and other inside organs.

The functions of an axial skeleton: Several essential activities are performed by the axial skeleton in the human body:
I. Protection: The cranium safeguards the brain, eyes, and auditory organs. The vertebral column envelops and safeguards the spinal cord. Within the thorax, the rib cage provides protection for the heart, lungs, and other essential physiological organs.
ii. Support: It serves as the primary structure that sustains the body's posture and preserves its overall structure. The spinal column bears the load of the head and trunk, enabling an erect body position.
iii. Movement: Although not principally responsible for movement, the axial skeleton serves as an attachment site for muscles that enable movement, including those important for breathing (intercostal muscles) and head and neck movement.
The vertebral column enables movement and flexibility of the torso, encompassing bending and twisting.

Haematopoiesis: The axial skeleton possesses red bone marrow, namely in the vertebrae, ribs, sternum, and pelvis, where the process of white blood cell formation (haematopoiesis) takes place.

i. Storage of minerals: The anatomical structures of the axial skeleton serve as reservoirs for vital minerals, including calcium and phosphorus, which may be released into the circulation as necessary to preserve mineral equilibrium.
ii. Location: Located within the skull, the bones of the middle ear (ossicles) are integral components of the axial skeleton and have a vital function in the transfer of sound from the outer ear to the inner ear, therefore facilitating the process of hearing.

Implications for clinical practice: A comprehensive knowledge of the axial skeleton is crucial in the medical domain for the identification and management of several disorders, including:
a. Fractures: Traumatic events can result in structural damage to the bones of the axial skeleton, notably in the vertebrae and ribs, necessitating urgent medical intervention.
b. Bone disorders: The vertebral column is often affected by spinal disorders such as scoliosis (an abnormal lateral curvature of the spine), herniated discs, and osteoporosis (a disease that weakens bones).

Arthritis refers to the degenerative alterations in the joints of the vertebral column, including osteoarthritis, which contribute to discomfort and restrict movement.
The axial skeleton can be impacted by infections such as osteomyelitis or diseased growths, including both benign and malignant types, requiring meticulous assessment and treatment.

Procedure:
I. Take the skeletal system carefully.
II. Do the physical examination (Inspection of parts of axial skeletal system):
a. Posture assessment: Observe the patient's standing and sitting posture to identify any abnormal curvatures (like scoliosis, kyphosis, or lordosis).
b. Skull examination: Check the skull for any asymmetry, deformities, or tenderness.
c. Spine inspection: Look for misalignment, muscle spasms, or abnormal movements in the spine.
i. Cervical Spine: Palpate for tenderness, muscle tightness, or misaligned vertebrae.
ii. Thoracic and Lumbar Spine: Palpate along the spinous processes to detect any abnormalities.
iii. Rib Cage: Palpate the ribs for tenderness, especially in cases of trauma to rule out fractures.
III. After completion of physical inspection put the skeletal system carefully from where you take it.

Observation: By knowing the parts of axial skeleton system the various bones present in it with its different size and shapes as well as the different functional activities and any deformities if its present.

Result: The axial skeleton system different parts of bones present in the central body was to be checked and studied.

Experiment Number – 05

Identification of appendicular bones.

Aim: To study the identification of appendicular bones.

References:
1.

2.

Requirements: Human skeletal system.

Theory:
The appendicular skeleton is the portion of the skeletal system that includes the side bones i.e., the limbs and the structures that attach them to the axial skeleton. It is primarily responsible for facilitating movement and interaction with the environment. The appendicular skeleton comprises 126 bones and is divided into the bones of the upper limbs, lower limbs, pectoral (shoulder) girdle, and pelvic girdle.

Structure of the Appendicular skeleton: The appendicular skeleton is structured into the subsequent anatomic categories:
I. The pectoral (shoulder) girdle (4 bones): An extensive range of motion is provided by the pectoral girdle, which connects the upper limbs to the trunk. It comprises two pairs of skeletal bones:

A. Clavicles (2 bones): The clavicles, sometimes referred to as collar bones, are elongated, S-shaped bones that are positioned horizontally across the front aspect of the thorax, superior to the first rib.
Functions: To provide as a support to maintain the scapula in place, therefore enabling the shoulder to have its full range of motion. In addition, the clavicles transfer mechanical force from the upper extremities to the central skeletal system.

B. Scapulae (2 bones): The scapulae, also known as shoulder blades, are planar, tripartite bones situated on the posterior aspect of the thoracic cage.

Characteristics are:
i. Glenoid cavity: An indentation of short depth that connects with the humeral head, creating the shoulder joint.
ii. Acromion: An osseous or bony extension that is anatomically linked to the clavicle.

iii. Coracoid process: A hook-like anatomical feature that serves as a point of attachment for the chest and arm muscles.

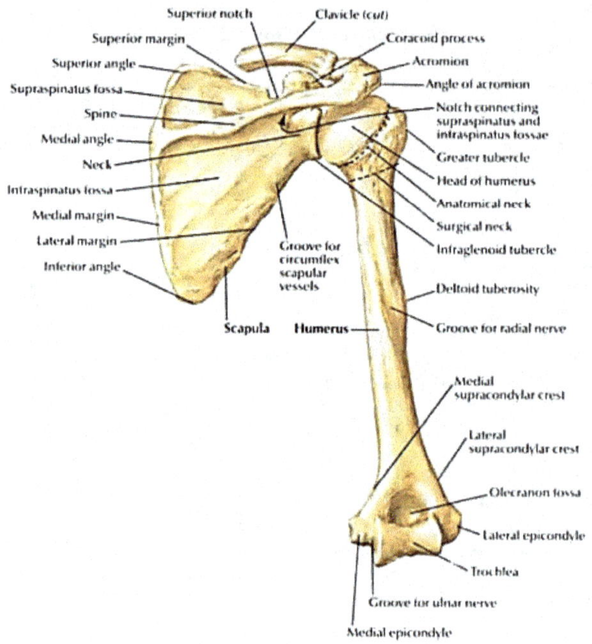

Fig. 5.1. Shoulder girdle

II. Upper limbs (60 bones):
Each upper limb consists of 30 bones, which are arranged into the arm, forearm, wrist, and hand.
A. Arm: (1 bone per limb): The humerus is the primary and most extensive bone in the upper extremity, stretching from the shoulder to the elbow.

Characteristics are:
i. The head is a conical anatomical formation that inserts into the glenoid cavity of the scapula, therefore constituting the shoulder joint.
ii. Deltoid tuberosity is a textured region where deltoid muscle attachment occurs.
iii. The distal end incorporates the trochlea and capitulum, which form articulations with the forearm bones.
iv. Forearm (2 bones per limb):

B. Radius is situated on the lateral aspect of the forearm, namely on the thumb side.
Characteristics: Rotation of the forearm (supination and pronation) is facilitated by the articulation of the head of the radius with the capitulum of the humerus.

C. Ulna: Situated on the inside aspects of the forearm.
Characteristics: Forming the prominence of the elbow, the olecranon process articulates with the trochlea of the humerus.

D. The wrist (carpus) consists of 8 bones per limb: A carpus is composed of eight tiny bones organized in two rows of four arrangements.

E. The proximal row consists of the scaphoid, lunate, triquetrum, and pisiform.

F. The distal row consists of the trapezium, trapezoid, capitate, and hamate. The bones confer or provide both flexibility and strength to the wrist.

G. Metacarpal bones (Each hand consists of 5 bones): The bones of the palm are individually numbered from I to V, commencing at the side of the thumb. Each hand consists of 14 phalanges, with the exception of the thumb, which contains two phalanges (proximal and distal), each finger consists of three phalanges (proximal, middle, and distal).

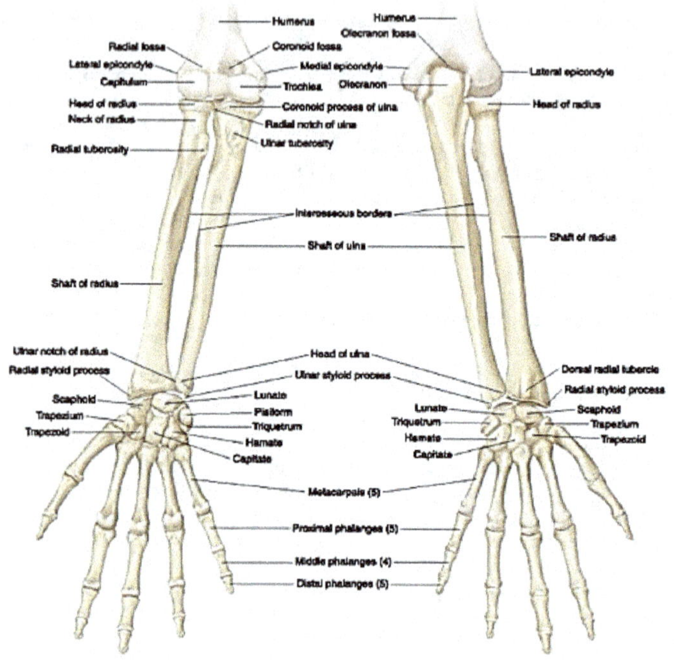

Fig. 5.2. Upper limbs.

III. Pelvic Girdle (consisting of 20 bones)

The pelvic girdle serves to immobilize the lower extremities to the central body and bear the load of the upper body. This structure comprises two hip bones, known as coxal bones, which are created by the fusion of three bones:

A. Ilium: The most extensive section of the hip bone, constituting the uppermost component.

Characteristics are: i. The iliac crest is the curving upper boundary, while the larger sciatic notch facilitates the transit of the sciatic nerve.

B. The ischium is the inferior, posterior section of the hip bone, The ischial tuberosity is a ridged region that supports weight during a seated position.

C. Pubis: The front part of the hip-bone.

Characteristics: A cartilaginous junction that units the two pubic bones is known as the pubic symphysis, upon convergence at the acetabulum, a deep socket, these three bones articulate with the head of the femur, therefore establishing the hip joint.

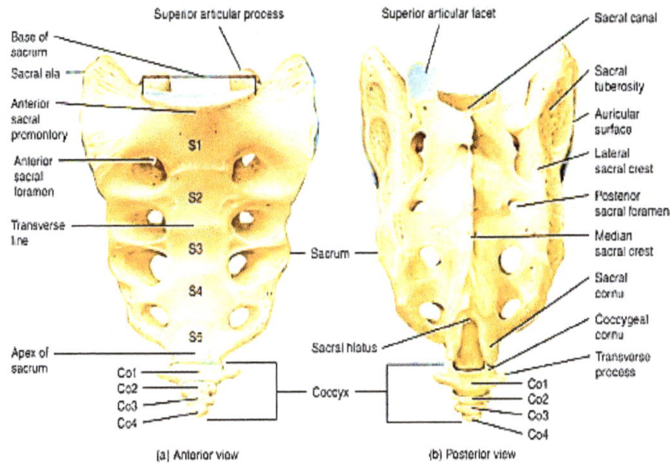

Fig. 5.3. Pelvic girdle.

IV. Lower Limbs (comprising 60 bones)

An individual lower limb consists of 30 bones, which are arranged into the thigh, leg, ankle, and foot.

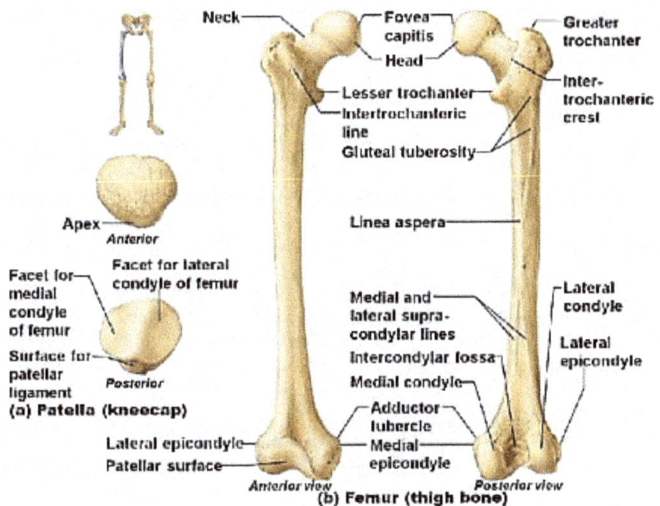

Fig. 5.4. Femur bone.

A. Thigh bone per limb: "The femur is the longest and most robust bone in the human body", stretching longitudinally from the hip to the knee. characteristics are:
i. The head forms the hip joint by articulating with the acetabulum of the pelvis.
ii. Neck: A very prone location for fractures, particularly among older persons.
iii. The distal end of the bone, which includes the medial and lateral condyles, articulates with the tibia.

B. Leg (2 skeletal bones per limb): The tibia is the bigger and more medial bone of the lower leg, responsible for supporting the majority of the body's weight.
Characteristic are:
i. The tibial tuberosity is its role as an attachment point for the patellar ligament.
ii. The fibula is a narrow bone situated laterally to the tibia.
iii. The fibula is a non-weight bearing structure that serves as a site for muscle attachment and contributes to the stabilization of the ankle.

C. Primary knee cap (1 bone per limb): The patella is a compact, triangular sesamoid bone that serves to safeguard the knee joint and provide the leverage to the quadriceps muscle.

D. The ankle (tarsus) consists of 7 bones per limb:
There are seven bones comprising the tarsus:
i. The talus articulates with the tibia and fibula to serve as the ankle joint.
ii. Calcaneus: The calcaneus, the heel bone responsible for supporting the body's weight.
iii. Additional skeletal structures consist of the navicular, cuboid, and three cuneiform bones (medial, middle, and lateral).

E. Foot:
i. Metatarsals: 5 bones per human foot, the bones that constitute the arch and ball of the foot are sequenced from the big toe side and numbered I to V.
ii. The phalanges consist of 14 bones in each foot. The bones of the toes, like the fingers, consist of three phalanges in each toe, except for the big toe which possesses two in arrangement.

Functions of Appendicular skeleton:
The appendicular skeleton performs many essential physiological roles, mostly associated with locomotion and engagement with the surroundings:
i. Movement: To facilitate movement, the appendicular skeleton offers leverage and places of attachment for muscles. The elongated rigid structures of the limbs function as levers, while the inter-articulations between these bones enable a broad spectrum of movement.
ii. Stabilization and equilibrium: The pelvic girdle bears the load of the upper body when standing and walking, while the foot arches facilitate the distribution of body weight across the foot, therefore serving to maintain balance.
iii. Protection: The bones of the appendicular skeleton provide protection for essential organs, for instance, the pelvis ensures the protection of organs within the pelvic cavity, whereas the shoulder girdle serves to screen the upper thorax.

iv. Mineralogical storage: Like the axial skeleton, the bones of the appendicular skeleton serve as repositories for vital minerals, including calcium and phosphorus.

v. In haematopoiesis: Haematological red bone marrow located in the long bones of the limbs serves as a location for the synthesis of blood cells, especially during growth and in situations of heightened need.

Significance in clinical settings: The appendicular skeleton is prone to a range of accidents, illnesses, and disorders:

i. Fractures are frequently seen in the appendicular bones as a result of falls, sports-related injuries, or accidents. In instance, the clavicle, radius, and femur are susceptible to fractures.

ii. Arthritis primarily impacts the joints of the appendicular skeleton, including the hips, knees, and shoulders, resulting in inflammation and limited range of motion.

iii. Dislocations: Traumatic injuries can cause dislocations in joints such as the shoulder or hip, necessitating immediate physician attention.

iv. Osteoporosis is a condition that weakens bones, significantly increasing their vulnerability to fractures, especially in the hips and wrists.

v. Developmental conditions such as hip dysplasia or clubfoot adversely impact the alignment and functionality of the appendicular bone from infancy.

<u>Procedure:</u>

I. Take the skeletal system carefully.

II. Do the physical examination (Inspection of parts of appendicular skeletal system):

a. Limbs: the upper and lower limbs each and every bone present in it, by its size and proper location.

b. Shoulder and pelvic girdles bones its size and the connecting linking parts with the appendicular to axial skeleton regions.

III. After completion of physical inspection put the skeletal system carefully from where you take it.

<u>Observation:</u> By knowing the parts of appendicular skeleton system the various bones present in it with its different size and shapes as well as the different functional activities and any deformities if its present.

<u>Result:</u> The appendicular skeleton system different parts of bones present other than the central body bones i.e., appendicular bones like limbs and girdle parts was to be checked and studied.

Experiment Number – 06

Introduction to hemocytometry.

Aim: To study the Hemocytometer.

References:
1.

2.

Requirements: Compound microscope, haemocytometer (Neubauer chamber).

Theory:
Hemocytometry is a method employed to quantify the number of cells, particularly blood cells, inside a certain volume of a fluid sample. This technique is crucial in clinical and scientific environments to quantify cell concentrations, including white blood cells (WBCs), red blood cells (RBCs), and platelets in the blood, as well as to enumerate additional cell types in biological preparations.

A. The fundamental concept of hemocytometry:
The principle behind hemocytometry is the direct microscopic enumeration of cells inside a predetermined volume. To achieve this objective, the haemocytometer, a specialized counting chamber, is employed. The chamber features a topographically engraved grid, upon which the sample is deposited. Quantifying the cell count within a specified region of the grid allows for the determination of cell concentration in the sample.

B. Structure of haemocytometer:
Quantification chamber: The haemocytometer is a glass slide of considerable thickness, including a central region that is gently indented to provide a chamber of a controlled depth, usually 0.1 mm.

Grid: Typically, the counting chamber is equipped with a pre-etched grid consisting of squares of predetermined proportions, such as 1 mm². Through the subdivision of the grid into smaller squares, precise and thorough counting is made possible. A specialized coverslip is positioned over the chamber to provide a consistent depth for the material under analysis.

C. Sample preparation:
In many cases, it is necessary to dilute the cell sample, such as blood, before counting to achieve adequate separation of the cells and enable subsequent precise counting.

Before loading into the haemocytometer, it is vital to meticulously mix the sample to guarantee uniform dispersion of cells.

Initial loading: A minute quantity of the diluted material is meticulously transferred into the counting chamber using a pipette. The material disperses by capillary action, filling the chamber devoid of any air bubbles.

D. Procedure for counting:
Microscope configuration: Orient the haemocytometer onto the microscope stage and fine-tune the focus. Utilize a low-power objective to identify the grid and thereafter transition to a higher-power objective for counting.

i. Cell counting: Determine the cell count in several grid squares, usually the four corner squares and the centroid square of a big grid. Only include cells that are completely contained inside the square or those that touch two of the borders (often the top and left) of the square to prevent duplicating the count.

ii. Quantification: The cellular concentration per unit volume is determined using the following formula:

Concentration of cells = Number of cells counted x Dilution factor/ the volume of the chamber counted.
The measured volume of the chamber is determined by the area of the grid squares and the corresponding depth of the chamber.

E. Applications:
i. Clinical haematology: Hemocytometry is employed to conduct comprehensive blood counts (CBC), which provide vital insights into the health status of a patient, encompassing counts of white blood cells (WBC), red blood cells (RBC), and platelets.
ii. Cell culture researchers utilize haemocytometers to quantify cells in culture for viability tests, and proliferation investigations, and to establish the optimal seeding density for laboratory procedures.
The technique of hemocytometry is employed in microbiology to quantify the number of bacterial cells or other microorganisms present in a given sample.

F. Limitations and considerations:
Ensuring accuracy in counting necessitates meticulous sample preparation, uniform distribution inside the chamber, and meticulous counting methodology. Inaccurate cell counts might result from errors in sample dilution, so it is important to ensure exact measurement and mixing.

Adherence to appropriate sample handling and preparation is necessary to prevent the presence of debris or clumping of cells, as these factors can disrupt precise counting.

G. Alternative approaches:
Although hemocytometry is a commonly used and dependable technique, automated cell counters and flow cytometry are alternative methods that provide quicker and frequently more precise cell counting, particularly in high-throughput environments.

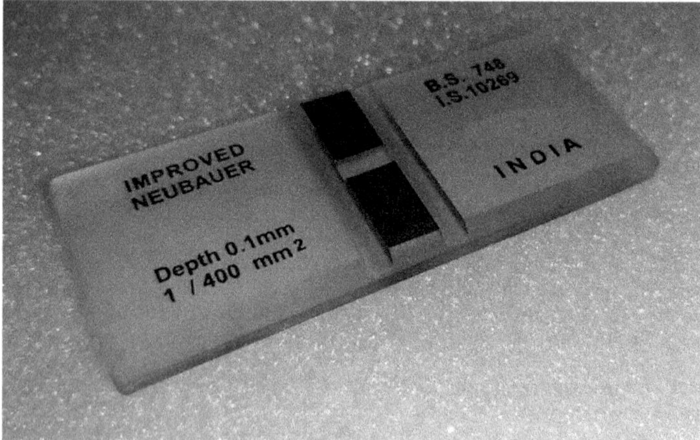

Fig. 6.1. hemocytometry (Neubauer chamber).

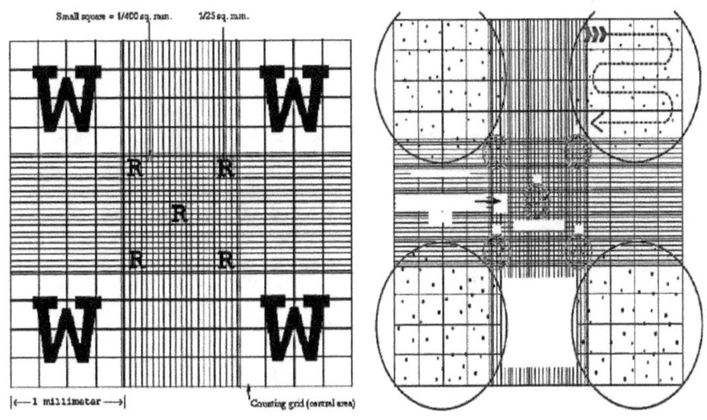

Fig. 6.2. The Neubauer chamber counts
(where W indicates "WBC" & R indicates RBC)

Procedure:

i. Take a clean and dry haemocytometer: Ensure it is clean and dry.

ii. Specialized Cover Slip: Use the cover slip provided with the haemocytometer to maintain a uniform chamber depth.

iii. Microscope: Set up a light microscope with appropriate magnification.

iv. Use Pipettes: Use a micropipette or capillary pipette to transfer the sample.

v. Dilution solution: If necessary, prepare a diluting fluid (e.g., saline or a specialized diluent depending on the cell type being counted).

vi. Sample: Have your cell sample (e.g., blood, cell suspension) ready.

vii.. Loading the haemocytometer: Place the Cover Slip: Carefully place the cover slip over the counting chamber of the haemocytometer.

viii. Pipette the sample: Use a pipette to draw up a small volume of the sample (usually 10-20 µL).

ix. Load the chamber: Touch the pipette tip to the edge of the cover slip and gently allow the sample to flow into the chamber by capillary action. The chamber should fill completely without air bubbles or overflowing.

x. Microscopic Counting: Set-up the Microscope and place the haemocytometer on the microscope stage, start with a low magnification (e.g., 10x objective) to locate the grid, then switch to a higher magnification (e.g., 40x) for counting.

xi. Record the Counts: Write down the number of cells counted in each square.

Calculate the cell concentration
Formula:
Cell Concentration (cells/mL) = Number of Cells Counted × Dilution Factor/ Volume of Chamber Counted.

xii. Cleaning and maintenance: Clean the haemocytometer after counting, carefully clean the haemocytometer and cover slip with distilled water and dry them with a lint-free tissue.

xiii. Store Properly: Store the haemocytometer and cover slip in a clean, dry place to prevent damage.

Observation: By checking the blood samples the WBC was to be checked at 40x magnification.

Result: The hemocytometry experiment was to be performed and the cell concentration was found to be________.

<u>Experiment Number – 07</u>

Enumeration of white blood cell (WBC) count.

Aim: To study the white blood cell (WBC) count.

References:
1.

2.

Requirements:
a. Instrument: Compound microscope, haemocytometer (Neubauer chamber).
b. Apparatus: Haemocytometer (Neubauer chamber), coverslip, micropipette.
C. Sample: Blood sample.

Theory:

White Blood Cells (WBCs), also known as leukocytes, are an essential component of the immune system, responsible for defending the body against infections, foreign invaders, and diseases. A WBC count is a common laboratory test used to measure the number of white blood cells in a given volume of blood. This count provides important information about a person's immune status and can help diagnose a variety of conditions.

I. Types of White blood cells:
a. Neutrophils: The most abundant type of WBC, responsible for responding quickly to infections, especially bacterial infections.
b. Lymphocytes: Includes T-cells, B-cells, and natural killer (NK) cells, which play a key role in the adaptive immune response.
c. Monocytes: These cells become macrophages and help in phagocytosis, engulfing and digesting pathogens and dead cells.
d. Eosinophils: Primarily involved in combating parasitic infections and allergic reactions.
e. Basophils: The least common type of WBC, involved in allergic reactions and releasing histamine during inflammatory responses.

II. Purpose of WBC count:
a. Infection detection: Elevated WBC counts often indicate the presence of an infection.
b. Immune system evaluation: Low WBC counts can indicate a compromised immune system, as seen in conditions like HIV/AIDS or bone marrow disorders.
c. Monitoring disease progression: WBC counts are monitored in diseases like leukemia, where abnormal increases or decreases in WBCs occur.
d. Response to treatment: WBC counts help assess how well a patient is responding to treatments such as chemotherapy or antibiotics.

III. Normal WBC count range:
a. The normal range for WBCs in adults is typically between 4,000 and 11,000 cells per microliter (cells/µL) of blood.
b. Leukocytosis: An elevated WBC count above 11,000 cells/µL, which can be caused by infections, inflammation, stress, or malignancies.
c. Leukopenia: A low WBC count below 4,000 cells/µL, which can be due to bone marrow suppression, severe infections, autoimmune disorders, or certain medications.

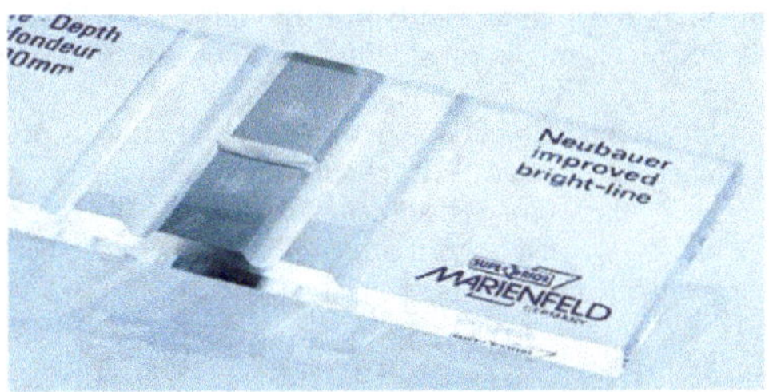

Fig. 7.1. Haemocytometer (Neubauer chamber) manual counting process.

IV. Methods for counting WBCs:
a. Manual counting using a haemocytometer: A blood sample is diluted and then loaded onto a haemocytometer. The number of WBCs within a defined grid area is counted under a microscope, this method requires careful technique and is less commonly used in clinical settings today due to the availability of automated counters.

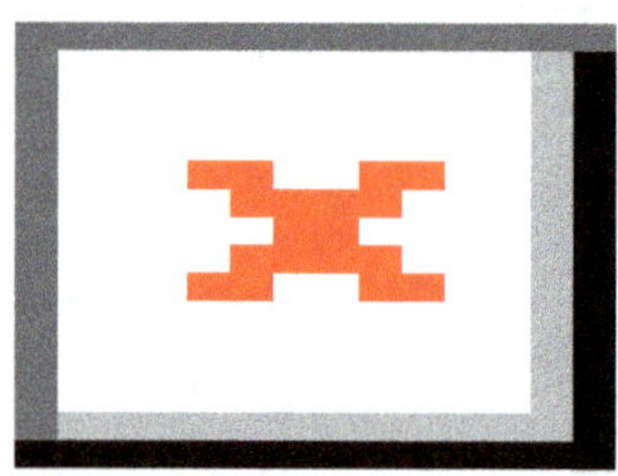

Fig. 7.2. Automated haematology analyser.

b. Modern laboratories typically use automated analyzers to count WBCs. These machines use principles like impedance or flow cytometry to rapidly count and differentiate WBCs with high accuracy.
Differential WBC Count: In addition to the total WBC count, a differential count is often performed to determine the proportion of each type of white blood cell. This provides more detailed information about the immune response and specific health conditions.

V. Clinical significance of WBC count:
i. Infections: A high WBC count is a typical response to bacterial infections. In contrast, viral infections might cause either an increase or decrease in WBC count, depending on the virus and stage of infection.
ii. Inflammatory disorders: Conditions like rheumatoid arthritis or inflammatory bowel disease can cause elevated WBC counts due to chronic inflammation.
iii. Leukemia and other blood disorders: Abnormal WBC counts can be indicative of leukemia or myelodysplastic syndromes, where the bone marrow produces abnormal white blood cells.

iv. Drug reactions: Certain medications, such as corticosteroids, can increase WBC counts, while others, like chemotherapy drugs, can suppress WBC production.

VI. Factors affecting WBC count:
a. Physical and Emotional Stress: Stress can temporarily increase WBC counts.
b. Medications: Steroids, antibiotics, and other drugs can affect WBC counts.
c. Smoking: Smoking can cause an increase in WBC counts due to the body's response to chronic irritation and inflammation.
d. Pregnancy: Pregnancy can lead to a slight increase in WBC counts, especially in the third trimester.

Procedure:

a. Take the Neubauer's chamber (Hemocytometer): Ensure it is clean and dry.
b. Specialized cover slip: Use the cover slip that comes with the haemocytometer to maintain a uniform chamber depth.
c. Microscope: Set up a light microscope with appropriate magnification 40x.
d. Pipettes: Use a micropipette or capillary pipette for transferring the sample and diluent.
e. Diluting fluid: Prepare an appropriate diluting fluid, such as Turk's solution (a common diluent for WBC counting), which lyses red blood cells and stains the WBCs for easy visualization.
f. Sample: Obtain a well-mixed blood sample, typically using an anticoagulated blood specimen (e.g., EDTA blood).
g. Dilute the Blood Sample: Dilute the blood sample at a standard ratio, commonly 1:20 or 1:100, depending on the expected WBC concentration, for mixing draw 0.1 mL of blood using a micropipette and mix it with 1.9 mL of Turk's solution in a clean test tube to achieve a 1:20 dilution.
h. **Loading the Neubauer's chamber and place the cover slip** carefully place the cover slip over the counting chamber of the hemocytometer.
i. Pipette the Diluted Sample: Use a pipette to draw up a small volume of the diluted blood sample (typically 10–20 µL), load the chamber by touching the pipette tip to the edge of the cover slip and gently allow the sample to flow into the chamber by capillary action. Ensure the chamber fills completely without air bubbles or overfilling.

Calculation:

WBC Count (cells/µL) = Number of WBCs Counted × Dilution Factor/ Volume of the Counting Area

Observation: By checking the blood samples the WBC was to be checked at 40x magnification.

Result: The white blood cell (WBC) count was found to be _______cells/ul.

<u>Experiment Number – 08</u>

Enumeration of total red blood corpuscles (RBC) count.

<u>Aim:</u> To study the total red blood corpuscles (RBC) count.

<u>References:</u>
1.

2.

<u>Requirements:</u>
a. Instrument: Compound microscope, haemocytometer (Neubauer chamber).
b. Apparatus: Haemocytometer (Neubauer chamber), coverslip, micropipette.

C. Sample: Blood sample.

Theory:
Red Blood Cells (RBCs), also known as erythrocytes, are the most abundant type of blood cell in the human body. They are responsible for transporting oxygen from the lungs to tissues and carbon dioxide from tissues back to the lungs. The total RBC count is a key haematological test that measures the number of red blood cells in a specific volume of blood. This count is crucial for diagnosing and monitoring various conditions, such as anaemia, polycythaemia, and other disorders affecting red blood cell production or destruction.

I. Structure and Function of RBCs

a. Shape: RBCs are biconcave, disc-shaped cells, which increases their surface area for oxygen exchange and allows them to deform as they pass through narrow capillaries.

b. Haemoglobin a protein that binds oxygen and gives red blood cells their characteristic colour, haemoglobin is essential for the transport of oxygen from the lungs to the rest of the body.

c. Lifespan: The average lifespan of an RBC is about 120 days, after which they are removed from circulation by the spleen.

d. **Oxygen Transport**: The primary function of RBCs is to carry oxygen. A sufficient number of RBCs is necessary to ensure that body tissues receive adequate oxygen.

e. Diagnosis: The RBC count helps diagnose conditions like anaemia (low RBC count) and polycythaemia (high RBC count). It also aids in evaluating hydration status, nutritional deficiencies, and bone marrow function.

f. Monitoring treatment: RBC counts are used to monitor the effectiveness of treatments for conditions affecting red blood cell production, such as chemotherapy, radiation therapy, or erythropoietin therapy.

g. Normal RBC Count Range

    i. Adult Males: 4.7 to 6.1 million cells per microliter (cells/μL) of blood.

    ii. Adult Females: 4.2 to 5.4 million cells/μL of blood.

    iii. Newborns and Children: Higher RBC counts are typically observed in newborns, which gradually decrease to adult levels.

h. Factors influencing RBC count:

    i. Physiological Factors: Age, sex, and altitude can affect RBC counts. For instance, people living at high altitudes often have higher RBC counts due to lower oxygen levels in the environment.

    ii. Pathological Factors: Conditions like anaemia (due to blood loss, iron deficiency, or bone marrow suppression), dehydration, and polycythaemia vera can lead to abnormal RBC counts.

    iii. Hydration Status: Dehydration can cause a relative increase in RBC count (haemoconcentration), while overhydration can dilute the blood and decrease the RBC count (haemodilution).

Methods for Counting RBCs:
A. Manual counting using a hemocytometry: A small sample of blood is diluted with an isotonic solution and loaded onto a haemocytometer (such as a Neubauer's chamber). The RBCs are then counted under a microscope in a defined grid area, and the total count is calculated.

B. Automated haematology analysers: In modern laboratories, automated analyzers are used to count RBCs. These machines use principles like electrical impedance or optical light scattering to quickly and accurately count RBCs in large numbers.

Procedure:

a. Take the Neubauer's Chamber (Hemocytometer): Ensure it is clean and dry.

b. Specialized Cover Slip: Use the cover slip that comes with the haemocytometer to maintain a uniform chamber depth.

c. Microscope: Set up a light microscope with appropriate magnification 80x.

d. Pipettes: Use a micropipette or capillary pipette for transferring the sample and diluent.

e. Diluting fluid: Diluting Fluid: Use an isotonic solution, such as Heyem's solution or Gower's solution, which preserves the shape of the RBCs without causing haemolysis.

f. Sample: Obtain a well-mixed blood sample, typically using an anticoagulated blood specimen (e.g., EDTA blood).

g. Dilute the Blood Sample: Dilution Ratio: Dilute the blood sample typically at a ratio of 1:200 to avoid overcrowding of cells on the haemocytometer, mixing and draw 0.02 mL (20 µL) of blood using a micropipette and mix it with 4 mL of the diluting fluid in a clean test tube to achieve a 1:200 dilution.

h. **Loading the Neubauer's chamber and place the cover slip** carefully place the cover slip over the counting chamber of the hemocytometer.

i. Pipette the diluted Sample: Use a pipette to draw up a small volume of the diluted blood sample (typically 10–20 µL), load the chamber by touching the pipette tip to the edge of the cover slip and gently allow the sample to flow into the chamber by capillary action. Ensure the chamber fills completely without air bubbles or overfilling.

Calculation:

RBC Count (cells/µL) = Number of RBCs Counted × Dilution Factor/
Volume of the Counting Area

Observation: By checking the blood samples the RBC was to be checked at 80x magnification.

Result: The Red blood cell (RBC) count was found to be _________ cells/ul.

<u>Experiment Number – 09</u>

Determination of bleeding time.

Aim: To study the bleeding time.

References:
1.

2.

Requirements:

a. Instrument: Stop watch.
b. Apparatus: Sterile pricking needle or lancet, blotting paper or filter paper.
C. Sample: Blood sample.

Theory:
Bleeding time is a diagnostic test used to quantify the duration required for a microvascular puncture to cease bleeding. It is a conventional technique employed to evaluate platelet function, platelet cell contacts with blood channel walls, and blood vessel constriction capacity. Despite the proliferation of more sophisticated assays, bleeding time remains valuable in specific clinical contexts for assessing primary haemostasis, the initial stage of the blood clotting process.

I. Objective of bleeding:
a. Evaluation of platelet activity: Bleeding time mainly characterizes the level of platelet functionality. Platelets are diminutive hematopoietic cells that have a pivotal function in the facilitation of coagulation to halt haemorrhaging. The test also offers indirect insights into the state of blood vessels, known as vascular integrity. Healthy blood arteries undergo constriction to facilitate haemostasis.
b. Screening for haemostatic disorders: The bleeding time test is employed to detect diseases associated with primary haemostasis, including von Willebrand disease, thrombocytopenia (low platelet count), and platelet function abnormalities.

II. Basis in physiology: Primary haemostasis refers to the process in which a blood artery responds to injury by constricting to decrease blood flow. Platelets subsequently attach to the visible wall of the blood artery, gather together to create a platelet block and secrete mediators that facilitate more blood clotting.

Platelet plug formation: The time it takes for a platelet plug to develop and halt bleeding shows the efficacy of primary haemostasis.

Vascular constriction refers to the capacity of blood arteries to narrow in reaction to damage, which in turn affects the duration of bleeding. Pathologies that hinder the narrowing of blood vessels might extend the duration of bleeding.

Normal bleeding time: It ranges from 2 to 7 minutes,
The presence of a prolonged bleeding period, over 7 minutes, indicates an impairment in platelet function, a reduced platelet count, or a concern with the integrity of blood vessels.

IV. Test indications:
i. A bleeding time test is recommended in cases when there is a suspicion of a platelet function abnormality or thrombocytopenia.
ii. Preoperative assessment: The test may be conducted preoperatively to evaluate the likelihood of severe haemorrhaging.
iii. Unexplained bleeding: This intervention is indicated for individuals who exhibit inexplicable bruises, nosebleeds, or persistent bleeding following small lacerations.

V. Bleeding time determination methods:

a. Duke's Methodology: An earlier technique involves creating a tiny incision on the earlobe or fingertip using a lancet. The duration required for bleeding to cease is documented. Today, this approach is less often utilized because of its inherent unpredictability.

b. Ivy's methodology: A conventional surgical cut is performed on the forearm using a specialized instrument, such as a Simplate or Surgicutt. Typically, the incision is 5 to 10 mm in length and 1 mm in depth.

The blood is thoroughly wiped using filter paper at 30-second intervals until bleeding ceases. The duration from the surgical cut to the point when bleeding stops is documented.

A revised version of Ivy's Method: Analogous to the Ivy technique, but with a quantified depth and length of the cut to enhance uniformity.

VI. Analysis of findings: Appropriate bleeding time is a key indicator of appropriate platelet function and sufficient constriction of blood vessels.

Prolonged bleeding time may suggest:

a. Thrombocytopenia is a condition characterized by a hypoplastic platelet count, typically caused by bone marrow abnormalities, autoimmune illnesses, or certain drugs.

b. Platelet dysfunction: Disorders such as von Willebrand disease or the use of medications that impact platelet function (e.g., aspirin, NSAIDs). Vascular Disorders: Distinct uncommon disorders that compromise the structural integrity of blood arteries, resulting in extended bleeding duration.

c. Variables influencing results: The administration of specific drugs, physiological circumstances (such as ambient temperature), and individual characteristics (such as age and skin type) of the patient might impact the duration of bleeding.

VII. Constraints of bleeding time variability: The duration of bleeding might be influenced by the methodology used by the examiner and the specific site of the cut.

Superseded by Contemporary Assessments: In light of its constraints, bleeding time has been mostly substituted by more precise diagnostic procedures, such as platelet function tests, PFA-100, and thromboelastographic.

Bleeding time is not indicative of all haemostatic malformations as it just evaluates primary haemostasis and does not include data on coagulation factors or secondary haemostasis, both of which are essential in the clotting process.

VIII. Clinical significance screening tool: Although possessing significant limits, bleeding time remains to be a valuable screening tool in specific contexts, particularly in areas with low resources where more sophisticated testing is not accessible. An atypical bleeding time result generally necessitates further testing to identify the root cause of abnormal haemostasis.

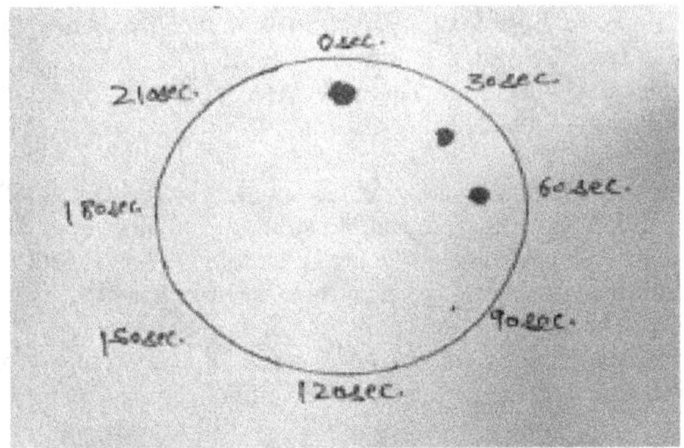

Fig. 9.1. Bleeding time.

Disorder caused by difference in clotting time:
A. Extended duration of bleeding: Extended bleeding duration suggests a prolongation in the formation of a platelet plug, sometimes caused by platelet malfunction or low platelet levels (thrombocytopenia), furthermore, it might arise from anomalies inside the blood vessels themselves.
i. Thrombocytopenia: It cause hypoplateletemia resulting in decreased platelet count in the bloodstream, causing compromised coagulation.
Symptoms: Allergic bruising, uncontrolled bleeding, epistaxis, periorbital haemorrhage, and extended bleeding from lacerations.

Idiopathic Thrombocytopenic Purpura (ITP) is an autoimmune condition characterized by the immune system actively attacking and eliminating platelets.
Aplastic Anaemia is a medical disorder characterized by inadequate production of blood cells, particularly platelets, by the bone marrow.

ii. Von Willebrand Disease (VWD) pathology: A hereditary condition resulting from an insufficiency or malfunction of Von Willebrand factor (VWF), a protein that facilitates platelet attachment to blood vessel walls and aids the activity of clotting factor-VIII.
Symptoms: Recurrent epistaxis, excessive menstrual cycles, proneness to bruising, and extended bleeding following traumas or surgical procedures.
Impact on bleeding time: Extended duration of bleeding caused by compromised platelet recruitment and development of blood clots.

iii. The Bernard- Soulier syndrome: A rare hereditary condition characterised by impaired platelet function caused by the lack or malfunction of the glycoprotein Ib/IX complex, essential for platelet attachment to the wall of blood vessels. presenting symptoms include prolonged bleeding, easy bruising, and frequent nosebleeds.
Bleeding time effect: markedly extended bleeding time caused by compromised platelet adhesion.

iv. Glanzmann Thrombasthenia: It causes an uncommon hereditary condition resulting from a lack of glycoprotein IIb/IIIa on the outer layer of platelets, essential for platelet aggregation.

Symptoms: Recurrent epistaxis, persistent gingival bleeding, proneness to bruising, and extended bleeding following traumas.
Impact on bleeding time: Extended duration of bleeding due to hindered aggregate formation of platelets.

v. Diffuse Ehlers-Danlos syndrome: It causes a collection of hereditary connective tissue diseases that impact the structural soundness of blood vessels, resulting in delicate blood vessels that are susceptible to spontaneous rupture.
Symptoms: Prone ecchymosis, recurrent haemorrhaging, excessive joint mobility, and erythematous or delicate skin.
Impact on bleeding time: Extended as a result of compromised blood vessel walls, resulting in heightened vulnerability to embolism.

vi. Uremia: It is a chronic kidney disease causes uremic toxins in individuals with renal insufficiency hinder platelet activity, resulting in extended bleeding durations.
Symptoms: Heightened susceptibility to spontaneous hemorrhage, facile bruising, and bleeding gums.
Impact on bleeding time: Extended duration of bleeding resulting from compromised platelet activity induced by the accumulation of toxins in the bloodstream.

vii. Drug induced prolonged bleeding: Haemorrhage of extended duration specific pharmaceutical medications can extend the duration of bleeding by disrupting platelet activity:
Aspirin acts as an inhibitor of the enzyme cyclooxygenase, therefore decreasing the synthesis of thromboxane A2, a mediator of platelet aggregation.
Non-Steroidal Anti-Inflammatory Drugs (NSAIDs) diminish platelet function. Clopidogrel and other oral antiplatelet medications: Suppress platelet aggregation, hence extending the duration of bleeding.
Symptoms: Extended haemorrhaging following lacerations, facile bruising, and epistaxis. Prolongation of bleeding time is attributed to decreased platelet aggregation.

ii. Reduced bleeding duration though uncommon, shortened bleeding time can arise in disorders characterized by abnormally increased clotting or platelet activity. Although not commonly linked to particular diseases, reduced bleeding time can suggest a hypercoagulable condition, characterized by an increased tendency of the blood to clot rapidly. Frequently, these illnesses coincide with thrombotic disorders, including:
a. Hypercoagulation: It cause the pathological states characterized by an increased the clotting time of blood to rapidly coagulate, hence increasing the risk of developing life-threatening blood clots (thrombosis). Potential causes may encompass:
b. Polycythaemia Vera is conditions characterised by excessive production of red blood cells and occasionally platelets, resulting in thicker blood and heightened risk of clotting.
c. Mutation of factor-V Leiden: An inherent genetic mutation that confers resistance to inactivation of Factor V, therefore resulting in heightened clot formation.

Symptoms: These disorders often do not result in symptoms of excessive bleeding, but they may manifest with signs of aberrant clot formation, such as deep vein thrombosis (DVT) or pulmonary embolism (PE).

Impact on the duration of bleeding: Increased clotting resulting in reduced or normal bleeding time.

Procedure:
1. Choose the correct finger (mostly the ring finger, middle finger, and index finger); cleanse the tip of the finger with spirit (with a concentration ranging from 60% to 95% alcohol) or any other acceptable wound antiseptic.
2. Perform a finger puncture using a sterile disposable needle to elicit unobstructed blood flow with minimal discomfort.
3. Promptly start the stopwatch and record the time.
4. After every 30 seconds, just touch the finger to absorb the blood drips by gently rubbing the puncture site on the filter paper without applying much pressure or squeezing the finger.
5. Assign sequential numbers to the bottom of the blood spots.
6. Record the moment bleeding ceases, namely when no remaining blood is stained on the filter paper.
7. The overall count of spots and record the number at which there is no presence of blood as the critical threshold.
8. State the outcome in units of minutes and seconds.

Observation: At this particular time up to _________minutes the bleeding spots stops and the time noted.

Result: The bleeding time of my blood was found to be ________ minutes.

<u>Experiment Number – 10</u>

Determination of clotting time.

Aim: To study the clotting time.

References:
1.

2.

<u>**Requirements:**</u>
a. Instrument: Stop watch.
b. Apparatus: Sterile pricking needle or lancet, both end open capillary.
C. Sample: Blood sample.

<u>**Theory:**</u>
Clotting time is the duration needed for blood to develop a stable clot, which stops more blood loss following an injury. Hematologic coagulation is an essential biological process characterized by a sequence of synchronized events, mostly involving blood arteries, platelets, and plasma proteins called clotting factors. A comprehensive elucidation of the clotting process, the associated pathways, and the variables influencing clotting time is provided here.

1. Introduction to haemostasis: Haemostasis is the physiological mechanism by which the body ceases uncontrolled bleeding at the specific location of an injury. The process has four primary stages:
a. Vascular spasm, also known as vasoconstriction, is the constriction of blood vessels to decrease blood flow to the affected anatomical region.
b. Formation of platelet plugs: Platelets attach to the exposed collagen of the damaged blood artery and arrange themselves into a transient plug.
c. cascade of coagulation: This is an intricate sequence of processes that result in the creation of a fibrin mesh, which serves to stabilize the platelet plug.
d. Haemostasis and disintegration of the blood clot following the formation of the clot, the body starts the process of mending and ultimately destroys the clot at the completion of healing.

2. The coagulation cascade: Pathways of inherent and external origin, the process of blood coagulation, or the production of clots, is facilitated by two interconnected routes: the intrinsic and extrinsic pathways. These pathways converge in a single pathway to finalize the clotting process, both routes include a sequence of enzymatic processes in which clotting factors (proteins) possess.

2.1 Intrinsic pathway:
a. Activation: Initiated by an injury occurring locally inside the blood vessel, interactions between factor-XII (Hageman factor) and exposed collagen or a negatively charged surface initiate the process.

b. Sequence:
i. Factor-XII (Hageman factor) undergoes activation to form factor-XIIa, It stimulates the conversion of factor-XI (Plasma thromboplastin antecedent) to factor-XIa, and then enzyme XIa converts factor-IX into its active form, factor-IXa (Christmas factor/ plasma thromboplastin component).
ii. By the interaction of calcium (Ca^{2+}) and factor-VIIIa (antihemophilic factor), factor-IXa stimulates the activation of factor-X (Stuart-prower factor). Compared to the extrinsic system, this pathway is characterized by a slower rate and a greater number of steps needed to commence the clotting process.

2.2 Extrinsic pathway activation: This pathway is activated by external damage that leads to the exposure of tissue factor, a protein concentrated in tissues located outside the blood vessels.

a. Chronology: In the bloodstream, tissue factor attaches to factor-VII (stable factor), therefore initiating its activation into factor-VIIa. The TF-VIIa complex stimulates the activity of factor-X (Stuart prower factor). This route exhibits superior speed and furnishes a more prominet reaction to vascular damage.

2.3 Shared pathway: Upon activation of factor-X, both the intrinsic and extrinsic routes converge. The common route comprises the subsequent stages:
a. The prothrombinase complex is formed by the combination of factor-X (Stuart prower factor), precipitated by either the intrinsic or extrinsic route, with factor-V (Labile factor), calcium ions, and phospholipids.
This complex enzymatically transforms factor-II prothrombin into thrombin. Subsequently, thrombin transforms fibrinogen factor-I into fibrin, which establishes a network that solidifies the blood clot.
Thrombin further stimulates factor-XIII, hence facilitating the cross-linking of fibrin strands to enhance the stability of the clot.

3. Contributing factors to clotting: Numerous clotting factors (proteins) and components are necessary for the effective development of a blood clot.
These include: Calcium ions (Ca^{2+}) function as a cofactor in several phases of the coagulation sequence. In the liver, vitamin K is necessary for the production of clotting factors-II (prothrombin), VII, IX, and X. Platelets release granules that supply supplementary components and function as a surface for the reactions as well. Clotting factors are assigned numerical values ranging from I to XIII, with the exception of factor-VI, which is independent of their function, individual factors have distinct roles in the coagulation cascade.

4. Stabilization and retraction of clots: Following the formation of fibrin strands, factor-XIII (fibrin-stabilizing factor) connects them together, resulting in a solid and durable clot that stops any excessive bleeding. Platelets subsequently undergo contraction, exerting force on the fibrin threads and therefore diminishing the dimensions of the clot, a phenomenon referred to as clot retraction, this contraction further acts to draw the borders of the incision closer together, therefore promoting the process of healing, upon reaching a sufficiently advanced stage of tissue healing, the clot is removed by a process known as fibrinolysis, mostly facilitated by the enzyme plasmin, which enzymatically breaks down fibrin into soluble pieces.

5. Variables Influencing clotting time: Determinants of blood coagulation time include genetic conditions, such as haemophilia (factor-VIII or IX deficiency), which can extend the time it takes for blood to clot because they hinder the production of blood clots, as the liver is the primary producer of clotting factors, illnesses such as cirrhosis can impact the process of coagulation.

Vitamin K deficiency: Vitamin K is necessary for the synthesis of certain tissue coagulation factors. Insufficient levels of it result in extended coagulation time.
In pharmaceutical medications like: Anticoagulants, such as heparin, warfarin, or aspirin, hinder several phases of the plasma coagulation process, therefore prolonging the time it takes for blood to clot.
Oral contraceptives can reduce serum clotting time by enhancing the synthesis of certain clotting components.

Hypoplateletemia (Thrombocytopenia): Impairs the body's capacity to generate a platelet plug, therefore extending the duration of bleeding and clotting.
Various environmental factors, including temperature and pH, might influence the speed of enzyme responses during the process of clotting.

6. Measurement of clotting time in clinical settings: A variety of laboratory assays are employed to quantify clotting time and evaluate coagulation function:
6.1. Test for clotting time: This is a fundamental test that quantifies the duration required for a blood sample to undergo coagulation. this procedure involves extracting blood and measuring the duration required for the development of a blood clot.

6.2 Prothrombin time (PT): The present test assesses the extrinsic route and the shared pathway of the coagulation cascade. The measurement quantifies the duration required for plasma to undergo coagulation subsequent to the introduction of tissue factor and calcium. The International Normalized Ratio (INR) is obtained from Procalcitonin and is employed for the purpose of monitoring patients who are taking anticoagulants such as warfarin.

6.3 Partial thromboplastin time (PTT): After activation the present test evaluates both the intrinsic pathway and the common pathway. This test quantifies the duration required for plasma to undergo coagulation following the introduction of an activator and calcium.

6.4 Thrombin-time (TT) analysis: This assay quantifies the percentage of fibrinogen that is converted into fibrin, therefore facilitating the detection of deficits in fibrinogen or the existence of thrombin inhibitors such as heparin.

6.5 Test for bleeding time: This assay is employed to assess platelet functionality and the structural soundness of tiny blood arteries; however, it does not directly quantify the duration of clotting.

7. Implications for clinical practice: A reduced clotting time suggests a propensity for excessive clot production, which may be caused by factors such as hypercoagulability, oral contraceptive usage, or the initial phases of disseminated intravascular coagulation (DIC), an extended clotting time indicates the presence of a bleeding condition, liver dysfunction, vitamin K insufficiency, or the impact of anticoagulant treatment such as warfarin or heparin.

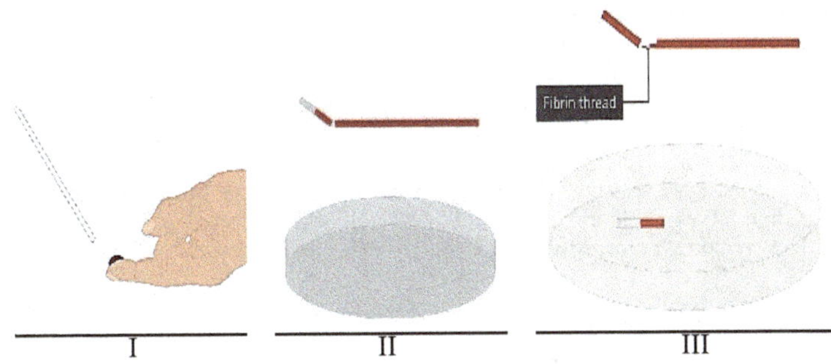

Fig. 10.1. Step involved in blood clotting time.

Disorder caused by difference in clotting time: Disorders caused by differences in clotting time are typically grouped into two major categories: bleeding disorders (where clotting time is extended) and clotting disorders (where clotting time is decreased, leading to increased clot formation). These abnormalities can emerge owing to inherited conditions, illnesses, medicines, or deficits in clotting factors.

A. Bleeding disorders (Prolonged clotting time): In certain situations, the blood takes longer to form a clot, resulting to heavy or persistent bleeding. Some common disorders include:

i. Haemophilia type: Genetic disease (X-linked recessive) causes haemophilia-A is due to a deficit of factor-VIII, and haemophilia-B (Christmas illness) is related to a shortage of factor-IX.

Symptoms: Prolonged bleeding, especially after injury or surgery, frequent nosebleeds, easy bruising, and internal bleeding (e.g., in joints).

Effect on clotting time: Clotting time is greatly delayed due to poor clotting factor activity.

ii. Von Willebrand Disease (VWD) Type: Genetic condition (autosomal dominant)

Cause: Deficiency or malfunction of Von Willebrand factor (VWF), a protein that helps platelets attach to injured blood arteries.

Symptoms: Prolonged bleeding from wounds, nosebleeds, severe menstrual bleeding, and bruises.

Effect on clotting time: Clotting time is lengthened, albeit frequently less significantly than in haemophilia, affects both platelet function and the clotting cascade.

iii. Disseminated Intravascular Coagulation (DIC) type: Acquired condition causes widespread activation of the clotting cascade, commonly induced by infections, trauma, malignancy, or severe inflammation. Initially, minute blood clots develop throughout the body, consuming clotting factors and platelets, resulting to a bleeding phase.

Symptoms: Excessive clotting followed by severe bleeding, organ failure, and shock.

Effect on clotting time: Clotting time increases lengthened as clotting factors and platelets are depleted.

iv. Liver disease type: Acquired condition causes liver to manufactures most clotting factors, hence liver illnesses such as cirrhosis, hepatitis, or liver failure can limit clotting factor production.
Symptoms: Easy bruising, bleeding from the gastrointestinal tract, and persistent bleeding following injury.
Effect on clotting time: Prolonged owing to reduced synthesis of clotting factors.

v. Vitamin-K deficiency type acquired condition causes vitamin-K is necessary for the creation of clotting factors-II, VII, IX, and X. Deficiency can arise owing to inadequate food intake, malabsorption, or usage of anticoagulants like warfarin.
Symptoms: Easy bruising, bleeding gums, nosebleeds, and persistent bleeding after surgery or trauma, effect on Clotting Time: Prolonged clotting time due to lower synthesis of vitamin K-dependent clotting factors.

vi. Thrombocytopenia type acquired or genetic cause low platelet count, which inhibits the development of the first platelet plug during haemostasis, causes might include autoimmune illnesses, bone marrow abnormalities, and certain drugs.
Symptoms: Easy bruising, persistent bleeding, and petechiae (small red or purple patches caused by bleeding into the skin).
Effect on Clotting Time: Prolonged due to the difficulty to produce a platelet plug.

B. Clotting Disorders (Shortened Clotting Time): In some situations, blood clots develop excessively fast, leading to excessive or aberrant clot formation (thrombosis). These clots can block blood arteries, producing serious consequences such as heart attacks, strokes, or deep vein thrombosis (DVT).

i. Factor-V Leiden type: Genetic condition cause mutation in factor-V, rendering it resistant to deactivation by activated Protein-C, a natural anticoagulant.
Symptoms: Increased chance of forming abnormal blood clots (thrombosis), especially in veins (DVT, pulmonary embolism).
Effect on Clotting Time: Clotting time is reduced or normal, but the danger of aberrant clot formation is greatly raised.

ii. Prothrombin Gene Mutation (G20210A) type: Genetic condition cause: A mutation in the gene for prothrombin (Factor-II) that leads to elevated quantities of this clotting factor.
Symptoms: Increased risk of blood clots in veins (DVT) or lungs (pulmonary embolism).
Effect on Clotting Time: Shortened clotting time due to higher prothrombin levels, resulting to quicker thrombin production.

iii. Antiphospholipid Syndrome (APS) Type: Autoimmune condition cause: The immune system develops antibodies that target phospholipids, which are critical components of cell membranes and play a role in the clotting process.

Symptoms: Recurrent blood clots, miscarriages, and strokes. APS can potentially lead to DVT, pulmonary embolism, or other problems owing to excessive clotting.

Effect on Clotting Time: Clotting time may be decreased, yet oddly, APS can occasionally extend clotting times in specific laboratory tests, despite the increased risk of clot formation.

iv. Hypercoagulability states type: Acquired or genetic cause: Conditions that enhance the chance of blood clotting. Causes might include cancer, pregnancy, obesity, surgery, and immobility.

Symptoms: Increased risk of blood clots in veins and arteries, leading to heart attacks, strokes, or pulmonary embolism.

Effect on clotting time: Clotting time may be normal or reduced due to an enhanced susceptibility for blood clot formation.

v. Oral contraceptive use and hormone replacement therapy type: acquired condition cause: Estrogen in birth control pills or hormone replacement treatment might boost the synthesis of specific clotting factors, making the blood more prone to clotting.

Symptoms: Increased risk of developing venous thromboembolism (VTE), including DVT and pulmonary embolism.

Effect on Clotting Time: Clotting time may be reduced, increasing the likelihood of aberrant clot formation.

vi. Polycythaemia vera type genetic condition cause: Excessive synthesis of red blood cells (and possibly platelets), resulting to thicker blood and an increased risk of clotting.

Symptoms: Headaches, dizziness, increased risk of blood clots, and flushed skin.

Effect on Clotting Time: Clotting time may be decreased due to increased blood viscosity and platelet numbers.

Procedure:

1. Choose the correct finger (mostly the ring finger, middle finger, and index finger); cleanse the tip of the finger with spirit (with a concentration ranging from 60% to 95% alcohol) or any other acceptable wound antiseptic.

2. Get a finger prick using sterile disposable needle to collect free flowing blood with minimum discomfort.

3. Immediately, start the stopwatch and note the time.

4. Touch one end of capillary tube towards the ozzes out blood, the blood will rise in tube via capillary action which may be augmented by retaining its open end at a lower level.

5. Note the time when blood starts to enter the capillary tube as zero time.

6. Hold the capillary tube between the palms of your hands to maintain the blood near body temperature.

7. Gently break off roughly 1 cm portions of capillary tube from one end at intervals of 30 seconds and examine for creation of fibrin thread of minimum 5 mm length between the broken ends of capillary tube. This is termed as rope formation. Note the time.

(Note: The average bleeding duration is 3-6 minutes).

Observation:
a. Name:
b. Age:
c. Gender:
d. Date:
e. Time of pricking:

Observation table:

S. No.	Timing of breaking capillary pieces	Formation of fibrin thread (yes/No)
1.	00:30	No
2.	01:00	No
3.	01:30	No
4.	02:00	No
5.	02:30	No
6.	03:00	No
7.	03:30	Yes

The fibrin thread was formed in capillary tube at time 03:30 minutes

Result: The clotting time of blood was found to be _________min.

<u>Experiment Number – 11</u>

Estimation of haemoglobin content.

<u>**Aim:**</u> To study the haemoglobin content.

<u>References:</u>
1.

2.

<u>Requirements:</u>
a. Instrument: Sahali's haemoglobinometer.
b. Apparatus: Sterile pricking needle or lancet.
C. Sample: Blood sample.

<u>Theory:</u>
Haemoglobin is a protein present in red blood cells (RBCs) that is important for the transportation of oxygen from the lungs to tissues and the retrieval of carbon dioxide from tissues back to the lungs for expiration. It is a vital constituent of blood, important for sustaining oxygen delivery and enabling cellular respiration.

A. The molecular structure of haemoglobin: The protein haemoglobin is a globular protein composed of four polypeptide chains arranged in a quaternary configuration. The association of each chain with a heme-group is characterized by the presence of an iron atom capable of binding a single oxygen molecule. Haemoglobin consists of two distinct categories of polypeptide chains: A pair of alpha (α) chains, Dual beta (β) chains, adult haemoglobin (HbA) is a tetramer composed of two α chains and two β chains, where each chain is folded into a condensed arrangement.

i. The heme group: Haemoglobin's heme group is a prosthetic group consisting of ferrous iron (Fe^{2+}) located in the centre of a big, ring-like organic molecule known as porphyrin.
Each iron ion inside a heme group forms a bond with a single oxygen molecule (O_2). Thus, each haemoglobin molecule has the capacity to bind a maximum of four oxygen molecules.

ii. Electrochemical oxygen binding and release reversibility characterizes the binding of oxygen to haemoglobin. Under conditions of high oxygen concentration in the lungs, haemoglobin combines with oxygen to produce oxyhaemoglobin, under conditions of low oxygen concentration in tissues, haemoglobin liberates oxygen for cellular use, transforming back into deoxyhaemoglobin.

B. Role of haemoglobin:
i. Transport of oxygen: The oxygen transfer from the lungs to tissues is significantly facilitated by haemoglobin, in the lungs, haemoglobin forms complexes with oxygen, resulting in a high partial pressure of oxygen of around 100 mm Hg. The release of oxygen by haemoglobin occurs as blood flows to tissues where oxygen is utilized and the partial pressure decreases to roughly 40 mm Hg.

C. Mechanisms of carbon dioxide transport:
Although the bulk of carbon dioxide (CO_2) is transported in the plasma as bicarbonate, haemoglobin also facilitates CO_2 translocation. Only a minute proportion of CO_2 directly attaches to haemoglobin, resulting in the formation of carbaminohaemoglobin, which is subsequently sent back to the lungs.
i. Buffering function: Haemoglobin functions as a buffer by attracting hydrogen ions (H^+) generated during metabolic activities, therefore assisting in the regulation of blood pH.

D. Classification of haemoglobin:
In humans, there are several forms of haemoglobin, which are determined by the developmental stage or genetic variances.
i. Haemoglobin A (HbA) is the main class of haemoglobin found in adults, accounting for approximately 95-98% of the total haemoglobin. constituted by a pair of α-globin chains and a pair of β-globin chains.
ii. Haemoglobin F (HbF) is the predominant variant of haemoglobin found in foetuses, consisting of two α-globin chains and two gamma (γ) chains. The affinity of HbF for oxygen is greater than that of HbA, therefore enabling the foetus to efficiently take oxygen from the mother blood.
iii. Haemoglobin A2 (HbA2) Constitutes around 2-3% of the overall haemoglobin
content in adults.
Composed of two chains of α-globin and two chains of delta (δ) subunits.
iv. Deviant haemoglobin parameters: The haemoglobin S (HbS) variant, present in persons with sickle cell disease, induces a sickle shape in red blood cells (RBCs), resulting in inadequate oxygen supply and obstructions in blood arteries. Haemoglobin C (HbC) is an additional aberrant form that can result in moderate hemolytic anemia.

E. Quantification of haemoglobin content:
Blood haemoglobin concentration is a significant clinical parameter quantified in grams per decilitre (g/dL). Haemoglobin levels in the normal range differ according to age, sex, and general health.
Adult males: 13.8 to 17.2 g/dL
Range for women: 12.1 to 15.1 g/dL
Kids: 11 to 16 grams per decilitre
Newborns: 14 to 24 g/dL

F. Haemoglobin measurement methods: There exist several techniques employed for the determination of haemoglobin concentration:
The cyanmethaemoglobin method involves the conversion of haemoglobin to cyanmethaemoglobin by the addition of potassium cyanide. The concentration is

subsequently determined by spectrophotometry. The haemoglobinometer is a basic instrument used to quantify the concentration of haemoglobin in blood by the use of light absorption methods. Automated blood analyzers are contemporary instruments employed in labs to quantify haemoglobin levels as a component of a comprehensive blood count (CBC).

G. Control of haemoglobin concentration:
i. Erythropoiesis: It is during erythropoiesis, the generation of red blood cells, that haemoglobin is synthesised. The control of this process which takes place in the bone marrow is contingent upon:
ii. Serum erythropoietin (EPO) is a renal hormone that triggers red blood cell (RBC) synthesis in reaction to hypoxia.
Elementary iron: A vital component in heme production. Anaemia can occur as a consequence of reduced haemoglobin synthesis caused by iron shortage. The presence of sufficient quantities of vitamin B12 and folate is essential for the appropriate maturation of red blood cells and the production of haemoglobin.

H. Haemoglobin content-related disorders:
i. Anaemia (Hyperglobinopathy): Anaemia is a condition characterized by decreased oxygen-carrying ability of the blood due to below-normal haemoglobin
levels.
Etiology of anemia encompasses:
a. Insufficiency of iron: The most prevalent kind of anemia is a result of insufficient iron levels required for the synthesis of haemoglobin.
b. Pernicious anemia: Characterised by a lack of vitamin B12, which hampers the synthesis of red blood cells.
c. Aplastic anemia is a medical disorder characterized by insufficient production of red blood cells by the bone marrow.
d. Sickle cell anemia is a condition characterized by the presence of aberrant haemoglobin (HbS) which alters the morphology of red blood cells, therefore diminishing their capacity to transport oxygen.
e. Thalassemia is a hereditary condition characterised by decreased or nonexistent biosynthesis of one of the globin chains, resulting in an unbalanced generation of haemoglobin, Thalassemia refers to a collection of hereditary conditions characterised by a diminished synthesis of either alpha or beta globin chains, resulting in haemoglobin imbalance and inefficient red blood cell generation. As a consequence, anemia occurs and in severe instances, regular blood transfusions become necessary.

ii. Polycythemia (Elevated haemoglobin content): Polycythemia is a condition characterised by high quantities of haemoglobin, resulting in increased viscosity of the blood. This condition may manifest as:
a. Primary polycythemia (Polycythemia Vera) is a syndrome of the bone marrow characterised by an over production of red blood cells.
b. Secondary polycythemia is a condition characterized by elevated erythropoietin production due to causes such as residing at high altitudes, chronic lung illness, or tumors that generate anthracycline (EPO).

iii. Haemoglobinopathies: Haemoglobin diseases are hereditary conditions resulting from abnormalities in the globin genes, which induce aberrant structure or function of haemoglobin. A mutation in the beta-globin gene results in the synthesis of HbS, which induces the stiffening and sickle-shaped formation of red blood cells, therefore obstructing blood arteries and diminishing oxygen supply.

I. Affinity of haemoglobin and oxygen: There are various variables that govern the capacity of haemoglobin to bind and release oxygen: In the lungs, when the partial pressure of oxygen (pO_2) is elevated, haemoglobin forms complexes with oxygen.

At decreasing pO_2 levels in tissues, haemoglobin liberates oxygen. The Bohr Effect is a phenomenon where an elevation in carbon dioxide levels and acidity (lower pH) reduces the affinity of haemoglobin for oxygen, therefore facilitating extracellular oxygen release in tissues. 2,3-Bisphosphoglycerate (2,3-BPG) is synthesised in erythrocytes and attaches to haemoglobin, reducing its affinity for oxygen and hence activating the release of oxygen in tissues.

Temperature: Elevated temperatures decrease the level of oxygen affinity of haemoglobin, therefore facilitating the transportation of oxygen during exercise.

J. Significance of haemoglobin content in clinical settings: Effective monitoring of haemoglobin levels is essential for the diagnosis and treatment of certain medical disorders:

a. Anaemia: The detection of reduced haemoglobin levels aids in the diagnosis of various forms of anemia and the monitoring of their therapy. In cases of polycythemia vera, persistent hypoxia, or tumors that produce erythropoietin, increased haemoglobin levels may be indicative of the presence of these disorders.

Diagnostic testing for atypical haemoglobin types enables the detection of disorders such as sickle cell disease and thalassemia, therefore facilitating timely intervention.

Haemoglobin levels can vary depending on age, sex, and other physiological parameters. The standard reference ranges for haemoglobin concentration, as determined by the Sahli's haemoglobinometer, are as follows:

i. The approximate range for adult males is 13.5 to 17.5 grams per decilitre (g/dL).

ii. In adult females, the serum glucose levels range from 12.0 to 15.5 g/dL.

iii. In children, the normal range can exhibit significant variation, usually ranging from 11.0 to 16.0 g/dL, contingent upon the age and growth stage of the kid.

Low haemoglobin levels: A low haemoglobin count, often indicative of anemia, can result from various conditions, including nutritional deficiencies (like iron or vitamin B12), chronic diseases, or bone marrow disorders. Symptoms of low haemoglobin may include fatigue, weakness, and shortness of breath, as the body struggles to deliver adequate oxygen to tissues.

High haemoglobin levels: Elevated haemoglobin levels can occur due to factors such as chronic hypoxia (low oxygen levels), dehydration, or conditions like polycythemia vera. High haemoglobin may not always present symptoms, but it can increase the risk of complications like blood clots

Clinical significance: Regular monitoring of haemoglobin levels is crucial, especially in patients with conditions that affect red blood cell production or destruction. Abnormal haemoglobin levels can indicate underlying health issues that may require further investigation or treatment.

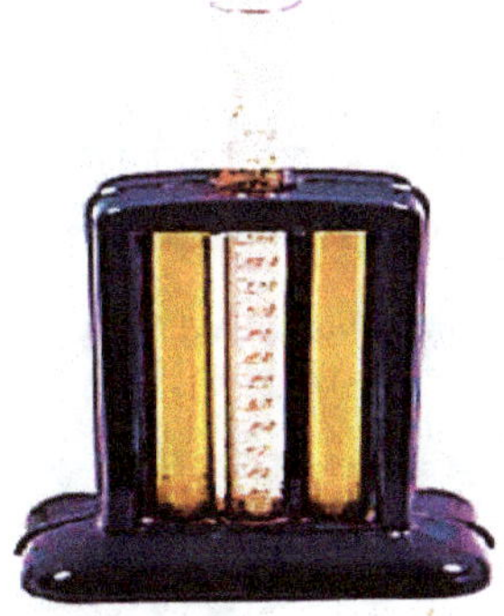

Fig. 10.1. Sahli's haemoglobinometer

Procedure: Haemoglobin content by using Sahli's haemoglobinometer.
1. Equipment preparation: Acquire the essential equipment i.e., haemoglobinometer, haemoglobin pipette, stirrer, and comparator tube manufactured by Sahli.
2. Verify that you have prepared N/10 hydrochloric acid and distilled water for immediate use.
3. Collection of samples: The haemoglobin pipette should be used to extract a minute volume of blood, typically 20 µl, from the patient.
4. Acidic mixing: Thoroughly cleanse the haemoglobin pipette by repeatedly drawing in and expelling the hydrochloric acid to guarantee its cleanliness.
5. Introduce the blood sample into the acid contained within the pipette. This combination will transform haemoglobin into acid hematin, a protein with a dark brown coloration.
6. Incubation period: The combination should be left undisturbed for approximately 10 minutes. The waiting interval is critically important as it enables
the most possible conversion of haemoglobin to acid hematin.
7. Dilution: Proceed to pour the mixture into the haemoglobinometer tube following the incubation period, add distilled water incrementally, drop by drop, until the color of the solution corresponds to that of a reference brown glass comparator.
8. Reviewing the outcome: Upon achieving colour matching, proceed to directly measure the haemoglobin value from the scale on the haemoglobinometer. Grams per deciliter (g/dL) is the usual unit of expression for this number.

Observation:
Name:
Age:
Gender:
Date:

Result: The haemoglobin content was found to be '…………' g%.

Experiment Number – 12

Determination of blood group.

Aim: To study the determination of blood group.

References:
1.

2.

Requirements:
a. Apparatus: Sterile pricking needle or lancet, glass slide.
b. Sample: Blood sample.
c. Chemical: Antisera (A, B & D).

Theory:
The determination of blood group refers to identifying the type of blood based on specific antigens present on the surface of red blood cells (RBCs). Blood group testing is crucial for blood transfusions, organ transplants, and pregnancy to ensure compatibility and prevent adverse immune reactions.

Major blood group systems:
i. ABO blood group system:
Based on the presence or absence of antigens A and B on the surface of RBCs.
Blood groups: A, B, AB, and O.
Group A: A antigens on RBCs and anti-B antibodies in plasma.
Group B: B antigens on RBCs and anti-A antibodies in plasma.
Group AB: Both A and B antigens on RBCs; no antibodies in plasma.
Group O: No A or B antigens on RBCs; both anti-A and anti-B antibodies in plasma.
Rh Blood group system: Based on the presence (Rh-positive) or absence (Rh-negative) of the D antigen.

This further classifies blood as A+, A-, B+, B-, AB+, AB-, O+, O-.
Methods of Blood Group Determination:
a. Forward Typing: Involves mixing a blood sample with antibodies against A and B antigens. If agglutination (clumping) occurs with anti-A antibodies, the

blood is type A; with anti-B, it's type B. No agglutination indicates blood type O, and clumping with both anti-A and anti-B shows AB.

Reverse typing: Tests the plasma (serum) of the blood sample for antibodies. The plasma is mixed with known A and B RBCs. Agglutination of A cells indicates the presence of anti-A antibodies (hence, type B blood), while agglutination of B cells indicates anti-B antibodies (type A).

Rh typing: A blood sample is mixed with anti-Rh (anti-D) serum. Agglutination indicates Rh-positive blood, while no reaction means Rh-negative.
Importance of blood group determination:
Transfusions: Receiving the wrong blood type can lead to severe immune reactions, where the body attacks the transfused blood.
Pregnancy: Incompatibility between the mother's and the fetus's Rh factor can cause hemolytic disease of the newborn (HDN).
Organ Transplants: Matching blood types helps prevent rejection of the transplanted organ.
Crossmatching: This is a more detailed compatibility test performed before a blood transfusion. It ensures that the donor's and recipient's blood do not react negatively when mixed.

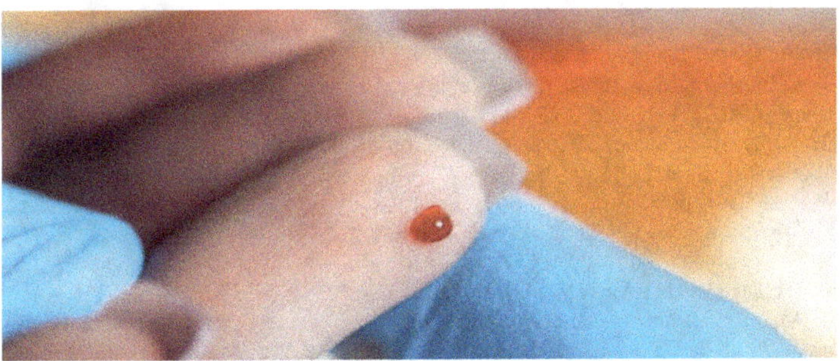

Fig 11.1. Blood group.

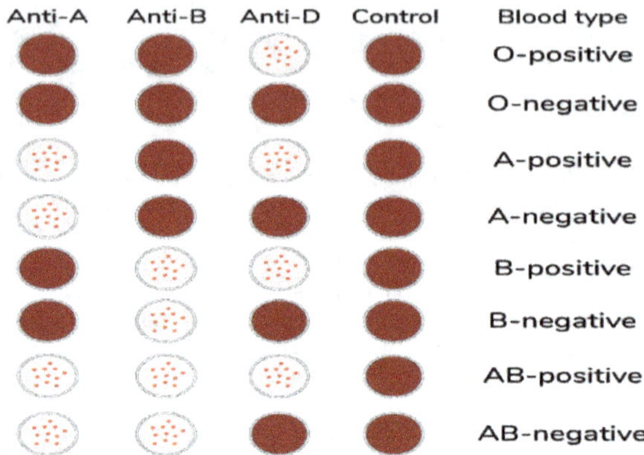

Table. 11.1. Blood group testing chart.

Procedure:

1. Label the slides: Label three sections of a glass slide or separate wells on a microplate as A, B, and D (Rh).

2. Apply blood sample: Place a small drop of the blood sample on each labelled section (A, B, and D).

3. Add Reagents:

i. To section A: Add a drop of Anti-A serum.

ii. To section B: Add a drop of Anti-B serum.

iii. To section D (Rh): Add a drop of Anti-D serum.

4. Mix the samples: Using separate mixing sticks (or toothpicks), gently mix each blood sample with its corresponding serum (Anti-A, Anti-B, and Anti-D) on the slide. Ensure that the samples are mixed thoroughly but avoid contaminating one section with another.

Observation:

A. For agglutination (Clumping): After mixing, observe the reactions for agglutination (clumping) of the red blood cells. This can be done visually or under a microscope for more detailed observation. For ABO Blood Group (A and B sections): Agglutination in section A only: Blood group A (A antigens present, anti-B antibodies in plasma). Agglutination in section B only: Blood group B (B antigens present, anti-A antibodies in plasma). Agglutination in both A and B sections: Blood group AB (both A and B antigens present, no antibodies). No agglutination in either section A or B: Blood group O (no A or B antigens, both anti-A and anti-B antibodies in plasma).

For Rh Factor (D section): Agglutination in section D: Rh positive (D antigen present). No agglutination in section D: Rh negative (no D antigen).

Confirm with Reverse Typing (Optional): Reverse typing can be done by mixing the patient's plasma with known A and B cells to confirm the presence of anti-A or anti-B antibodies. Agglutination with A cells indicates blood group B (presence of anti-A antibodies). Agglutination with B cells indicates blood group A (presence of anti-B antibodies). No agglutination in both indicates blood group AB. Agglutination in both indicates blood group O.

Result: Blood group analysis was performed and my blood group was found to be _______________.

Experiment Number – 13

Determination of erythrocyte sedimentation rate (ESR).

Aim: To study the determination of erythrocyte sedimentation rate (ESR).

References:
1.

2.

Requirements:
a. Apparatus: Sterile pricking needle or lancet, Westergren-Katz tube.
b. Sample: Blood sample.
c. Chemical: EDTA

Theory:
Determination of Erythrocyte Sedimentation Rate (ESR): Erythrocyte Sedimentation Rate (ESR) is a common haematology test that measures how quickly red blood cells (erythrocytes) settle at the bottom of a test tube in a given period of time, typically one hour. ESR is an indirect measure of inflammation in the body. It's often used to diagnose and monitor diseases like infections, cancers, and autoimmune disorders.

Purpose of the Test:
The ESR test helps in:

i. Detecting inflammation or infection.

ii. Monitoring the progress of diseases like rheumatoid arthritis, tuberculosis, and autoimmune disorders.

iii. Determining the severity of conditions like temporal arteritis and polymyalgia rheumatica.

Principle of ESR: When anticoagulated blood is allowed to stand in a vertical tube, red blood cells settle due to gravity. The rate at which they settle depends on various factors, particularly the protein composition of plasma. In cases of inflammation, the concentration of acute phase proteins like fibrinogen increases, which causes the red blood cells to form stacks (rouleaux formation). These stacked red cells settle faster than individual cells, resulting in a higher ESR.

Methods for ESR determination: There are two common methods for measuring ESR: Westergren method (Standard method) and Wintrobe method (Less commonly used)

1. Westergren method (most widely used method):
Materials required: Westergren tube (200 mm long, 2.5 mm internal diameter)
Westergren stand
Anticoagulant (3.8% sodium citrate or EDTA)
Blood sample (venous blood)
Timer (for 1 hour)

Procedure:
i. Blood collection: Collect venous blood in a tube containing an anticoagulant (sodium citrate in 4:1 ratio of blood to anticoagulant).
ii. Filling the Westergren Tube: Mix the anticoagulated blood sample well.
Fill the Westergren tube up to the 0 mark (zero mark) with the anticoagulated blood.
iii. Placing the tube in a stand: Place the filled tube vertically in a Westergren stand. Ensure the tube is stable and upright.
iv. Incubation for 1 Hour: Allow the tube to stand undisturbed at room temperature for 1 hour. Make sure the environment is free from vibrations and temperature fluctuations, as they can affect the test results.
v. Reading the ESR value: After 1 hour, measure the distance from the top of the plasma (clear, yellowish liquid) to the top of the sedimented red blood cells. The result is expressed in millimeters per hour (mm/hr).

Normal ESR Values (Westergren method):
Men: 0-15 mm/hr
Women: 0-20 mm/hr
Children: 0-10 mm/hr
Newborns: 0-2 mm/hr
In conditions like infections, autoimmune diseases, and malignancies, ESR can be significantly elevated.

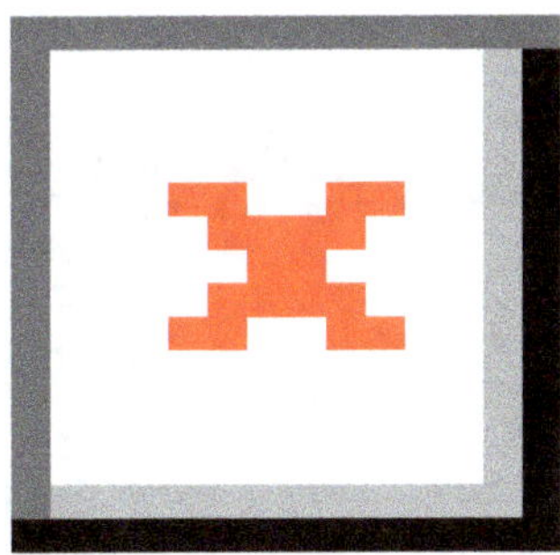

Fig.13.1. Westergren-Katz tube.

2. Wintrobe method:
Materials required: Wintrobe tube (shorter than Westergren tube, 100 mm in length), anticoagulated blood (EDTA)

Procedure:
i. Blood collection: Collect venous blood in an EDTA tube (commonly used as the anticoagulant for the Wintrobe method).
ii. Filling the tube: Fill the Wintrobe tube to the 0 mark with the blood sample.
iii. Placing the tube vertically: Place the Wintrobe tube vertically in a stand and leave it undisturbed for 1 hour.
Reading the ESR Value:
After 1 hour, measure the distance in millimeters from the top of the blood column to the top of the sedimented erythrocytes.

Normal ESR Values (Wintrobe method):
Men: 0-9 mm/hr
Women: 0-20 mm/hr
Factors Affecting ESR:
Increased ESR: Inflammation, infections, anemia, pregnancy, autoimmune diseases (e.g., lupus, rheumatoid arthritis), malignancies (e.g., multiple myeloma).
Decreased ESR: Polycythemia, sickle cell disease, hyperviscosity, and heart failure.
Clinical Significance of ESR:

High ESR: May indicate conditions such as tuberculosis, chronic kidney disease, systemic lupus erythematosus (SLE), rheumatoid arthritis, and malignancies.
Low ESR: May occur in polycythemia (excess red blood cells), leukocytosis, or congestive heart failure.
Normal ESR: Doesn't necessarily rule out disease, especially in early stages of inflammation.

Observation: The sedimentation of blood was observed, higher ESR values indicate a faster rate of erythrocyte sedimentation, which can suggest inflammation or disease (e.g., infections, autoimmune disorders, or cancers).

Result: The Erythrocyte sedimentation rate (ESR) was to be studied.

<u>Experiment Number – 14</u>

Determination of heart rate and pulse rate.

<u>**Aim:**</u> To study the heart rate and pulse rate.

<u>**References:**</u>
1.

2.

<u>**Requirements:**</u> Human-being.

<u>**Theory:**</u>
Heart rate and pulse rate are important physiological indicators of the body's cardiovascular function. Both terms are closely related but not identical. The heart rate refers to the number of times the heart beats per minute, while the pulse rate refers to the number of palpable arterial pulses per minute, which is a reflection of the heart's contractions.

Objectives:

To understand the difference between heart rate and pulse rate.
To learn how to measure heart rate and pulse rate manually and using instruments.
To interpret the significance of heart rate and pulse rate in health and disease.
What is heart rate?
Heart rate is the number of times the heart contracts (beats) per minute (bpm). The heart pumps blood throughout the body, delivering oxygen and nutrients to tissues and removing carbon dioxide and other waste products. The heart rate varies based on physical activity, emotions, body temperature, and overall health.

Normal heart rate:
Adults: 60-100 bpm (at rest)
Athletes: 40-60 bpm (at rest)
Newborns: 100-160 bpm
What is pulse rate?
Pulse rate refers to the number of palpable pulses of the arteries per minute, which are caused by the rhythmic pumping of the heart. When the heart contracts, blood is ejected from the left ventricle into the arteries, creating a wave of increased pressure (pulse) that can be felt at various points on the body.

Common pulse points:
Radial artery (at the wrist)
Carotid artery (in the neck)
Brachial artery (inner elbow)
Femoral artery (in the groin)
Popliteal artery (behind the knee)
Dorsalis pedis artery (top of the foot)
In most cases, heart rate and pulse rate are the same. However, in some pathological conditions, such as arrhythmias or heart failure, the heart may contract without effectively pumping blood, resulting in a difference between the heart rate and pulse rate (called a pulse deficit).

Relationship between heart rate and pulse rate:
Normally, the heart rate (number of heartbeats) equals the pulse rate (number of arterial pulsations).
Any discrepancy between the two is termed a pulse deficit, and this may occur due to irregular heart rhythms like atrial fibrillation.
Measuring heart rate:
Heart rate can be measured by manually feeling the pulse or using electronic devices such as heart rate monitors or ecg machines.

1. Manual method:
Radial pulse measurement (at the wrist): a. Place the index and middle fingers on the inside of the wrist (just below the thumb).
b. Gently press until you feel the pulse.
c. Count the beats for 30 seconds, then multiply by 2 to get the heart rate in bpm (beats per minute).
d. Ensure the person is at rest for accurate readings.

Carotid pulse measurement (at the neck): a. Place your index and middle fingers gently on one side of the neck, just beside the windpipe.
b. Press gently until you feel the pulse.
c. Count the beats for 30 seconds and multiply by 2.

2. Electronic devices:
a. Heart rate monitors: these are wearable devices (e.g., fitness trackers or chest straps) that measure heart rate using sensors that detect the electrical signals of the heart.
b. Electrocardiogram (ECG): this is the most accurate way to measure heart rate. ECG records the electrical activity of the heart over time, producing a waveform from which heart rate and rhythm can be analyzed.
c. Pulse oximeter: this device clips onto the finger and measures both pulse rate and oxygen saturation by detecting changes in blood flow.

Measuring pulse rate:
Pulse rate can be measured at various sites where arteries are close to the skin surface, and the pulse is palpable.
Common pulse sites:
i. Radial pulse: at the wrist, below the thumb.
ii. Carotid pulse: in the neck, next to the trachea.
iii. Brachial pulse: at the inner aspect of the arm, just above the elbow.
iv. Femoral pulse: in the groin.
v. Dorsalis pedis pulse: on the top of the foot.

Procedure for measuring pulse rate: a. Position the person: ensure the person is relaxed and seated or lying down.
b. Locate the pulse: use your index and middle fingers to palpate the artery at the chosen pulse site.
c. Counting the beats: Count the number of pulsations for 30 seconds and multiply by 2 for a pulse rate in bpm.
d. Count for 60 seconds for a more accurate reading if the pulse is irregular.

Factors affecting heart rate and pulse rate:
Age: children typically have higher heart rates than adults.
Fitness level: athletes often have lower resting heart rates.
Emotional state: stress, anxiety, and excitement can increase heart rate.
Medications: certain medications, such as beta-blockers, slow heart rate, while others, like stimulants, increase it.
Physical activity: exercise raises heart rate to meet the body's increased oxygen demand.
Temperature: fever can raise heart rate, while cold environments can slow it.

Clinical significance of heart rate and pulse rate:
1. Tachycardia (fast heart rate):
Heart rate > 100 bpm at rest is called tachycardia.
Causes include: Fever, anemia, hyperthyroidism, heart conditions such as arrhythmias, anxiety or stress, physical exertion
Certain medications (e.g., stimulants)
2. Bradycardia (slow heart rate):

Heart rate < 60 bpm at rest is called bradycardia.
Causes include: Well-trained athletes (normal physiological bradycardia), hypothyroidism.
Certain medications (e.g., beta-blockers)
Heart block or other cardiac conduction problems
3. Arrhythmias (irregular heart rate):
An irregular heart rate, where the heart may beat too fast, too slow, or with an abnormal rhythm.
Atrial fibrillation is a common type of arrhythmia, which can result in a pulse deficit (heart rate higher than the pulse rate).

Resting heart rate vs. Active heart rate:
Resting heart rate: measured when a person is at rest, usually in a seated or lying position. It reflects the efficiency of the cardiovascular system. A lower resting heart rate is often seen in athletes and indicates good cardiovascular fitness.

Active heart rate: measured during or immediately after exercise. It increases to supply muscles with more oxygenated blood. The heart rate during exercise can give an indication of cardiovascular endurance.

Observation: The heart rate and pulse rate are mostly affected by the influencing factors involved in it.

Result: The heart rate and pulse rate were to be studied and performed.

Experiment Number – 15

Recording of blood pressure.

Aim: To study the recording of blood pressure.

References:
1.

2.

Requirements:
a. Instruments: Stethoscope, sphygmomanometer.

Theory:
Blood pressure (BP) is the force exerted by circulating blood on the walls of blood vessels. It is one of the most important vital signs and helps assess cardiovascular health. Blood pressure is recorded as two numbers:

i. Systolic pressure: The pressure when the heart contracts and pumps blood into the arteries.
ii. Diastolic pressure: The pressure when the heart is at rest between beats.

Purpose of blood pressure measurement:
a. To diagnose conditions like hypertension (high blood pressure) and hypotension (low blood pressure).
b. To monitor patients with cardiovascular diseases or assess the risk of heart disease.
c. To check the effectiveness of treatments for high or low blood pressure.

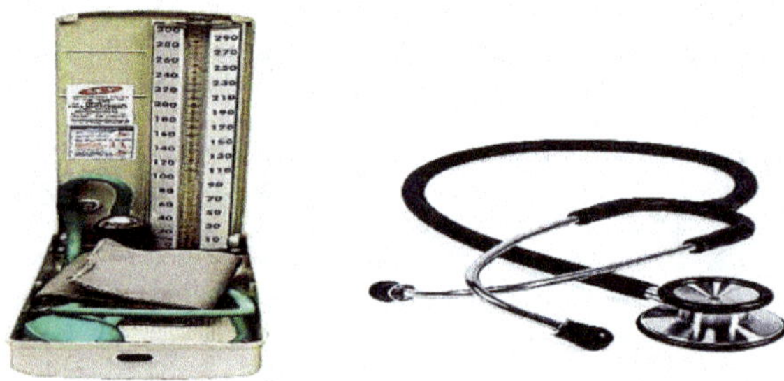

Fig. 15.1. Stethoscope and sphygmomanometer.

Instruments for measuring blood pressure:
There are two main instruments used for blood pressure measurement:
Sphygmomanometer (Manual or mercury-based) with digital blood pressure Monitor
1. Manual (Mercury or Aneroid) sphygmomanometer: This method involves the use of a stethoscope and a sphygmomanometer, which consists of an inflatable cuff, a pressure gauge, and a hand pump.
2. Digital blood pressure monitor: Digital monitors are more automated and provide systolic, diastolic, and pulse rate readings on a digital display. These monitors are easy to use but may not always be as accurate as manual readings.

Components of a Sphygmomanometer:
a. Inflatable cuff: Wraps around the upper arm to restrict blood flow.
b. Bulb pump: Used to inflate the cuff.
c. Pressure gauge: Measures the pressure in the cuff in millimeters of mercury (mmHg).
d. Stethoscope (manual method): Used to listen for Korotkoff sounds (arterial blood flow sounds) during the measurement.

Procedure for Blood Pressure Measurement (Manual Method):
1. Ensure the person is relaxed and has been seated for at least 5 minutes.

2. The arm should be at heart level, supported, and free of clothing.

3. The person should avoid exercise, caffeine, or smoking 30 minutes before the measurement.

4. Positioning the Cuff: Wrap the cuff snugly around the upper arm, about 2-3 cm above the elbow. The center of the cuff's bladder should be aligned with the brachial artery (on the inner side of the arm).

5. Inflating the Cuff and place the stethoscope diaphragm over the brachial artery (just below the cuff).

6. Close the valve on the bulb and inflate the cuff by squeezing the bulb until the gauge reads 20-30 mmHg above the expected systolic pressure (usually around 180 mmHg).

7. Deflating the Cuff and Listening for Korotkoff Sounds:

8. Slowly deflate the cuff by turning the valve on the bulb, allowing the pressure to drop at 2-3 mmHg per second.

9. Listen for the Korotkoff sounds: The first appearance of a rhythmic tapping sound corresponds to systolic pressure (first number).

As the pressure continues to drop, the sounds become muffled and eventually disappear. The point at which the sound disappears marks the diastolic pressure (second number).

10. Recording the measurement: Record both the systolic and diastolic pressures (e.g., 120/80 mmHg). Repeat the measurement on the other arm or wait a few minutes before repeating on the same arm to ensure accuracy.

Interpretation of blood pressure readings:

Normal Ranges for Adults:

Normal Blood Pressure: Less than 120/80 mmHg

Elevated Blood Pressure: Systolic between 120-129 and diastolic less than 80 mmHg

Hypertension (Stage 1): Systolic between 130-139 or diastolic between 80-89 mmHg

Hypertension (Stage 2): Systolic 140 mmHg or higher, or diastolic 90 mmHg or higher

Hypertensive Crisis: Systolic over 180 and/or diastolic over 120 mmHg (requires immediate medical attention)

Factors influencing blood pressure readings:

a. Position: Blood pressure can vary if the person is lying down, sitting, or standing.

b. Stress: Physical or emotional stress can elevate blood pressure.

c. Exercise: Blood pressure increases during physical activity.

d. Medications: Some drugs can raise or lower blood pressure.

e. Time of day: Blood pressure is typically lower in the morning and increases throughout the day.

f. Caffeine and Nicotine: Both can temporarily raise blood pressure.

Errors in Blood Pressure Measurement:

Cuff Size: Using an incorrect cuff size can lead to inaccurate readings (too small = high reading, too large = low reading).

Cuff Placement: Incorrect positioning of the cuff can affect the accuracy.

Inflation/Deflation Speed: Inflating or deflating the cuff too quickly can lead to errors in systolic and diastolic readings.

Talking or Moving: Movement or speaking during the measurement can alter results.

Procedure for digital blood pressure monitor:
1. Sit comfortably with the arm at heart level.
2. Relax for a few minutes and avoid speaking or moving during the measurement.
3. Positioning the Cuff: Place the cuff around the upper arm as per the device's instructions.
4. Starting the Device: Press the start button to inflate the cuff automatically.
5. The device will record the systolic and diastolic pressure, as well as the pulse rate, and display the readings on a screen.
6. Recording the Measurement: Note the readings and, if necessary, take multiple readings for accuracy.

Observation: The blood pressure was fluctuating depends on different factors involved.

Results: Blood pressure was to be studied and performed. My blood pressure was found to be normal 120/80.

<u>**Rough work page – I**</u>

<u>**Thank You.**</u>

www.ingramcontent.com/pod-product-compliance
Lightning Source LLC
LaVergne TN
LVHW010820200726

843507LV00003B/655